Sexual health, human rights and the law

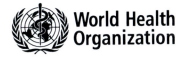

World Health Organization

WHO Library Cataloguing-in-Publication Data

Sexual health, human rights and the law.

1.Reproductive Health. 2.Human Rights. 3.Reproductive Health Services. 4.Sexuality. 5.Sex Offenses. 6.Social Responsibility. 7.Sexually Transmitted Diseases. 8.Legislation as Topic. I.World Health Organization.

ISBN 978 92 4 156498 4   (NLM classification: WQ 200)

Contents

Acknowledgements   v

Executive summary   1

I. Introduction   4

    1.1 Sexuality, sexual health and human rights   4

    1.2 Laws, human rights and their importance for sexual health   5

    1.3 Legal and policy implications   6

    II.Methodology and limitations   7

    2.1 Process   7

    2.2 Scope   7

    2.3 Search strategy and data sources   8

        2.3.1 Human rights, legal and jurisprudential data   8

        2.3.2 Public health data   9

    2.4 Critical assessment and synthesis of retrieved information   10

    2.5 Peer review and document preparation   11

    2.6 Limitations of the research and the report   11

III. Health services for the promotion and protection of sexual health   13

    3.1 Introduction   13

    3.2 Creating enabling legal and regulatory frameworks and eliminating barriers to services for sexual health   14

        3.2.1 Access to essential medicines   14

        3.2.2 Conscientious objection by health-care providers   15

        3.2.3 Availability and quality of health-care facilities and providers   15

        3.2.4. Criminalization of sexual-health-related services   16

    3.3 Ensuring quality and respect of human rights in the provision of sexual health services   16

        3.3.1 Guarantee of privacy and confidentiality   16

        3.3.2 Fostering informed decision-making   17

        3.3.3 Skilled health-care personnel   18

        3.3.4 Quality of supplies and equipment   18

    3.4 Elimination of discrimination in access to health services – addressing the specific needs of particular populations   18

        3.4.1 Adolescents (under 18 years of age)   19

        3.4.2 Marital status   20

        3.4.3 Incarceration   21

        3.4.4 Migrants and asylum seekers   21

        3.4.5 HIV status   22

        3.4.6 Disability   23

3.4.7 Sexual orientation and gender identity   23

3.4.8 Transgender and gender variant people   24

3.4.9 Intersex people   26

3.4.10 People engaged in sex work   27

3.5 Conclusion   29

3.6 Legal and policy implications   29

IV. Information and education for sexual health   31

4.1 Introduction   31

4.2 Defining sexuality information
and education   31

4.3 Legal restrictions on sexuality information and education   32

4.4 Human rights standards and legal protections   32

4.5 Ensuring no arbitrary or unnecessary restrictions to information and education related to sexuality
and sexual health for people under 18   33

4.6 Conclusion   34

4.7 Legal and policy implications   34

V. Sexual and sexuality-related violence   35

5.1 Introduction   35

5.2 Health, human rights and legal implications of different forms of sexual and sexuality-related violence   36

5.2.1 Sexual assault including rape   36

5.2.2 Sexual abuse of children   37

5.2.3 Forced marriage and sexual and sexuality-related violence   38

5.2.4. Violence based on real or perceived sexual behaviour or expression   40

5.2.5 Violence against people engaged in sex work   42

5.2.6 Trafficking for forced prostitution   43

5.2.7 Female genital mutilation   44

5.2.8 Coercive practices within health services that affect sexual health and sexuality   45

5.3 Conclusion   46

5.4 Legal and policy implications   46

References   48

Acknowledgements

The Department of Reproductive Health and Research of the World Health Organization (WHO/RHR) gratefully acknowledges the contributions that many individuals and organizations have made to the development of this report. We would particularly like to acknowledge the contribution of the following people to the development of this document:

Overall development: Jane Cottingham and Eszter Kismödi, former staff members of the WHO Department of Reproductive Health and Research; in partnership with Sofia Gruskin of the Program on Global Health and Human Rights, University of Southern California, Los Angeles, United States of America (USA); and Alice M. Miller, Global Health Justice Partnership of the Yale Law School and the School of Public Health, New Haven, USA.

Rajat Khosla coordinated the finalization of this report.

Legal research: Hossam Bahgat, Kajal Bhardwaj, Simone Cusack, Vivek Divan, Stefano Fabeni, Alice M. Miller, Charles Ngwena, Esteban Restrepo-Saldarriaga, Mindy Roseman and Johanna Westeson.

Additional contributors: Carolina Oyekanmi Brugat, Mauro Cabral, Sonia Correa, Erin Hetherington, Barbara Klugman, Alicia Peters, Stephanie Schlitt, Kristjana Sigurbjorndottir, Jaime Todd-Gher, Carol Vance and Gretchen Williams.

WHO staff: Avni Amin, Claudia García-Moreno, Rajat Khosla.

Development partners and funders: Ford Foundation, New York, USA; Open Society Institute, New York, USA; United Nations Development Programme.

Editing: Jane Patten of Green Ink, United Kingdom (greenink.co.uk)

Acronyms and abbreviations

CEDAW   Convention on the Elimination of All Forms of Discrimination against Women

CESCR   United Nations Committee on Economic, Social and Cultural Rights

DFID   United Kingdom's Department for International Development

GDG   Guideline Development Group

GRADE   Grading of Recommendations Assessment, Development and Evaluation

HIV   human immunodeficiency virus

ICPD   International Conference on Population and Development

IUD   intrauterine device

LARC   long-acting reversible contraception

MSI   Marie Stopes International

PBF   performance-based financing

PSI   Population Services International

SRH   sexual and reproductive health

UNFPA   United Nations Population Fund

USAID   United States Agency for International Development

WHO   World Health Organization

Executive summary

Sexual health today is widely understood as a state of physical, emotional, mental and social well-being in relation to sexuality. It encompasses not only certain aspects of reproductive health – such as being able to control one's fertility through access to contraception and abortion, and being free from sexually transmitted infections (STIs), sexual dysfunction and sequelae related to sexual violence or female genital mutilation – but also, the possibility of having pleasurable and safe sexual experiences, free of coercion, discrimination and violence. Indeed, it has become clear that human sexuality includes many different forms of behaviour and expression, and that the recognition of the diversity of sexual behaviour and expression contributes to people's overall sense of well-being and health.

Developments over the past three decades, particularly in the wake of the HIV pandemic, have brought an understanding that discrimination and inequality also play a key role in whether or not people can attain and maintain sexual health. For example, those who are perceived as having socially unacceptable sexual practices or characteristics, such as being HIV-positive, being an unmarried sexually active adolescent, a sex worker, a migrant, a transgender or intersex person, or engaging in same-sex sexual behaviour, suffer both marginalization and stigma, which take a huge toll on people's health. Those who are deprived of, or unable to access, information and services related to sexuality and sexual health, are also vulnerable to sexual ill health. Indeed, the ability of individuals to achieve sexual health and well-being depends on their access to comprehensive information about sexuality, knowledge about the risks they face, vulnerability to the adverse consequences of sexual activity, access to good quality sexual health care, and access to an environment that affirms and promotes sexual health. As well as being detrimental to their sexual health, discrimination and inequalities may also constitute a violation of human rights.

The achievement of the highest attainable standard of sexual health is therefore closely linked to the extent to which people's human rights – such as the rights to non-discrimination, to privacy and confidentiality, to be free from violence and coercion, as well as the rights to education, information and access to health services – are respected, protected and fulfilled. In the past two decades, an important body of human rights standards pertaining to sexuality and sexual health has been developed. This includes: interpretations by United Nations human rights treaty monitoring bodies of the content of human rights provisions; international, regional and national court decisions; international consensus documents; and reports by the United Nations Special Rapporteur on the Right to the Highest Attainable Standard of Health, among others. These standards are made operational through the enactment and implementation of laws, regulations and policies at the national level.

Laws matter because they set the rules of society and can provide the framework for the implementation of sexual-health-related policies, programmes and services. They can provide human rights guarantees, but they may also create limitations. Either way, laws and regulations have an impact on the enjoyment of the highest attainable standard of sexual health. Harmonizing laws with human rights standards can foster the promotion of sexual health across and within various populations, while the negative impact of laws that are in contradiction with human rights standards has been increasingly documented. For example, laws that foster the dissemination of objective, comprehensive sexuality information, if implemented for all, contribute to people's knowledge of what protects or damages their sexual health, including where and how to seek further information, counselling and treatment if needed. On the other hand, laws that restrict women's and adolescents' access to health services – for example, by requiring third-party authorization for services – and laws that criminalize certain consensual sexual behaviour can exclude or deter people from seeking and receiving the information and services they require and to which they have a right.

This report demonstrates the relationship between sexual health, human rights and the law. Drawing from a review of public health evidence and extensive research into human rights law at international, regional and national levels, the report shows how states in different parts of the world can and do support sexual health through legal and other mechanisms that are consistent with human rights standards and their own human rights obligations. This executive summary presents a few examples selected from the numerous examples provided in the full report.

Removal of legal and regulatory barriers to services

Ill health related to sexuality is vast and represents a significant disease burden throughout the world, so that access to appropriate health services for the wide range of sexual health problems is essential. At the same time, the right to the highest attainable standard of health has been defined and elaborated as encompassing a variety of facilities, goods and services that must be available, accessible, acceptable and of good quality. These are dimensions that have yet to be fulfilled in many places, and frequently this is due to an inadequate legal framework, including direct legal barriers. Among a number of examples of legal barriers to access is the prohibition or restriction on the availability of emergency contraception or on the delivery of services by health-care personnel other than doctors. In a number of countries this has been challenged and modified to make essential medicines and services available.

How services are provided

Because issues related to sexuality and sexual practices concern people's private lives and may be considered sensitive in many contexts, the guarantees of privacy, confidentiality and informed decision-making, for example, in the delivery of services, are particularly important. Where these guarantees are lacking, people may simply not use the services they need, with negative consequences for their health. Adolescents, for example, often avoid seeking services when confidentiality is not guaranteed and where parental authorization is required. Recognizing the importance of this dimension, and reflecting human rights standards, some countries have enshrined the guarantees of privacy, confidentiality and informed decision-making in law.

Access to information and education

Access to information and education relating to sexuality and sexual health is essential to enable people to protect their health and make informed decisions about their sexual and reproductive lives. Evidence shows that access to such information – as well as to comprehensive sexuality education that provides not only information but also builds personal communication skills – is associated with positive health outcomes. Laws and regulations that exclude specific topics from sexuality information and education, or exclude certain people from gaining access to sexuality education, have detrimental consequences for sexual health.

International human rights bodies have emphasized the importance of states providing sexuality information and comprehensive sexuality education for both adults and adolescents, and have specifically stipulated that states should refrain from censoring scientifically accurate sexual health information, or withholding or intentionally misrepresenting health-related information, including sexual education and information. Some states have promulgated laws that make specific provision for sexuality information and education through the right to education; in others, the restriction on information regarding abortion services, for example, has been successfully challenged at the regional level.

The use of criminal law

All legal systems use criminal law to deter, prosecute and punish harmful behaviour, and to protect individuals from harm. However, criminal law is also applied in many countries to prohibit access to and provision of certain sexual and reproductive health information and services, to punish HIV transmission and a wide range of consensual sexual conduct occurring between competent persons, including sexual relations outside marriage,

Executive summary

Sexual health today is widely understood as a state of physical, emotional, mental and social well-being in relation to sexuality. It encompasses not only certain aspects of reproductive health – such as being able to control one's fertility through access to contraception and abortion, and being free from sexually transmitted infections (STIs), sexual dysfunction and sequelae related to sexual violence or female genital mutilation – but also, the possibility of having pleasurable and safe sexual experiences, free of coercion, discrimination and violence. Indeed, it has become clear that human sexuality includes many different forms of behaviour and expression, and that the recognition of the diversity of sexual behaviour and expression contributes to people's overall sense of well-being and health.

Developments over the past three decades, particularly in the wake of the HIV pandemic, have brought an understanding that discrimination and inequality also play a key role in whether or not people can attain and maintain sexual health. For example, those who are perceived as having socially unacceptable sexual practices or characteristics, such as being HIV-positive, being an unmarried sexually active adolescent, a sex worker, a migrant, a transgender or intersex person, or engaging in same-sex sexual behaviour, suffer both marginalization and stigma, which take a huge toll on people's health. Those who are deprived of, or unable to access, information and services related to sexuality and sexual health, are also vulnerable to sexual ill health. Indeed, the ability of individuals to achieve sexual health and well-being depends on their access to comprehensive information about sexuality, knowledge about the risks they face, vulnerability to the adverse consequences of sexual activity, access to good quality sexual health care, and access to an environment that affirms and promotes sexual health. As well as being detrimental to their sexual health, discrimination and inequalities may also constitute a violation of human rights.

The achievement of the highest attainable standard of sexual health is therefore closely linked to the extent to which people's human rights – such as the rights to non-discrimination, to privacy and confidentiality, to be free from violence and coercion, as well as the rights to education, information and access to health services – are respected, protected and fulfilled. In the past two decades, an important body of human rights standards pertaining to sexuality and sexual health has been developed. This includes: interpretations by United Nations human rights treaty monitoring bodies of the content of human rights provisions; international, regional and national court decisions; international consensus documents; and reports by the United Nations Special Rapporteur on the Right to the Highest Attainable Standard of Health, among others. These standards are made operational through the enactment and implementation of laws, regulations and policies at the national level.

Laws matter because they set the rules of society and can provide the framework for the implementation of sexual-health-related policies, programmes and services. They can provide human rights guarantees, but they may also create limitations. Either way, laws and regulations have an impact on the enjoyment of the highest attainable standard of sexual health. Harmonizing laws with human rights standards can foster the promotion of sexual health across and within various populations, while the negative impact of laws that are in contradiction with human rights standards has been increasingly documented. For example, laws that foster the dissemination of objective, comprehensive sexuality information, if implemented for all, contribute to people's knowledge of what protects or damages their sexual health, including where and how to seek further information, counselling and treatment if needed. On the other hand, laws that restrict women's and adolescents' access to health services – for example, by requiring third-party authorization for services – and laws that criminalize certain consensual sexual behaviour can exclude or deter people from seeking and receiving the information and services they require and to which they have a right.

same-sex sexual behaviour and consensual sex work. The criminalization of these behaviours and actions has many negative consequences for health, including sexual health. Persons whose consensual sexual behaviour is deemed a criminal offence may try to hide it from health workers and others, for fear of being stigmatized, arrested and prosecuted. This may deter people from using health services, resulting in serious health problems such as untreated STIs and unsafe abortions, for fear of negative reactions to their behaviour or health status. In many circumstances, those who do access health services report discrimination and ill treatment by health-care providers.

International human rights bodies have increasingly called for decriminalization of access to and provision of certain sexual and reproductive health information and services, and for removal of punishments for HIV transmission and a wide range of consensual sexual conduct occurring between competent persons. National courts in different parts of the world have played an important role in striking down discriminatory criminal laws, including recognizing the potentially negative health effects.

Gender identity and expression

Being able to determine and express one's gender identity without stigma, discrimination, exclusion and violence is an important dimension of health and well-being and the enjoyment of human rights. The possibility for people to live in accordance with their self-identified gender, in law and in fact, has a beneficial effect on their overall well-being, including being able to access health, social and other services. The respect, protection and fulfilment of human rights require that no one should be forced to undergo medical procedures, including gender-affirming surgery, sterilization or hormone therapy, or be forced to divorce, as a requirement for legal recognition of their gender identity and expression. A number of national laws that previously required such procedures for a change of identity have been challenged and modified, or new laws have been promulgated, to be in line with human rights standards.

Sexual and sexuality-related violence

All forms of sexual and sexuality-related violence have multiple negative effects on health and well-being. People living in violent relationships, for example, may be unable to make sexual and reproductive choices, either through direct exposure to forced or coerced sex or because they are unable to control or negotiate regular use of contraception and condoms. This puts them at risk of unwanted pregnancy (for women), and STIs including HIV. Intimate partner violence in pregnancy increases the likelihood of abortion, miscarriage, stillbirth, preterm delivery and low birth weight.

An example of the way in which the law has an impact on sexual health is the legal understanding of rape, which has historically been understood as sexual intercourse by a man with a woman who is not his wife, through force and against her will, involving vaginal penetration by a penis. Under such a definition, women who have been raped by their husbands, women who have been raped anally, men and transgender individuals cannot claim, legitimately, to have been raped. International criminal law has evolved to define rape in much broader terms, covering different invasive acts perpetrated by and against people of any sex or gender, and recognizing that rape within marriage is a crime in all circumstances. Many national laws have been amended over the past decade in line with these human rights standards. This accommodates access to needed health services for all (unmarried girls and women, men, boys and transgender persons) as well as recourse to due process and redress, which plays a role in health.

Conclusion

States have obligations to bring their laws and regulations that affect sexual health into alignment with human rights laws and standards. Removing barriers in access to sexual health information and services, and putting in place laws and regulations that aim to support and promote sexual health, are actions that are also in line with the World Health Organization's global reproductive health strategy adopted by the World Health Assembly in 2004.

I. Introduction

Sexual health is fundamental to the physical and emotional health and well-being of individuals, couples and families, and ultimately to the social and economic development of communities and countries. However, the ability of individuals to achieve sexual health and well-being depends on them having: access to comprehensive information about sexuality; knowledge about the risks they face and their vulnerability to the adverse consequences of sexual activity; access to good quality sexual health care; and an environment that affirms and promotes sexual health (1). National laws and policies, both those governing the provision of health services (including information and education) and criminal, civil and administrative laws that are applied to sexuality-related matters, play a key role in fostering or hindering sexual health, and in promoting and protecting people's human rights related to sexual health.

This report explains and discusses the relationship between sexual health, human rights and the law. Drawing from a review of public health evidence and extensive research into human rights law at international, regional and national levels, the report demonstrates how states in different parts of the world can and do support sexual health through legal and other mechanisms that are consistent with human rights standards and their own human rights obligations. The report is directed at policy-makers in the field of health, health-care providers, nongovernmental organizations (NGOs) and others concerned with the promotion of sexual health and human rights. It seeks to help governments and policy-makers improve sexual health through bringing their laws and policies into alignment with national and international human rights obligations.

1.1 Sexuality, sexual health and human rights

Sexual health was first defined in a World Health Organization (WHO) Technical Report series in 1975 as "the integration of the somatic, emotional, intellectual and social aspects of sexual being, in ways that are positively enriching and that enhance personality, communication and love" (2). Twenty years later, the Programme of Action of the International Conference on Population and Development (Cairo, 1994) included sexual health under the definition of reproductive health, indicating that its purpose "is the enhancement of life and personal relations, and not merely counselling and care related to reproduction and sexually transmitted diseases" (3). While the mention of sexual health was important in this context, subsuming it under reproductive health meant that all the dimensions of sexuality and sexual health that go beyond reproduction were given less attention in subsequent programmes and policies.

Yet the past three decades have brought dramatic changes in understanding of human sexuality and sexual behaviour. The HIV pandemic has played a major role in this, but it has not been the only factor. The toll taken on people's health by other sexually transmitted infections (STIs), unwanted pregnancies, unsafe abortion, infertility, sexual violence and sexual dysfunction has been amply documented and highlighted in national and international studies and declarations (4).

During the same period, there has been a rapid increase in the documentation and understanding of the nature of discrimination and inequality related to sexuality and sexual health. This includes information about the marginalization, stigmatization and abuse of those perceived as having socially unacceptable sexual practices or characteristics (e.g. being HIV-positive, engaging in same-sex sex, being a sexually active adolescent, a sex worker, a transgender or intersex person, or any combination of these), and the toll that such discrimination takes on people's health. Many documented cases involve violations of human rights, such as the rights to health, life, equality and non-discrimination, privacy, and to be free from inhuman and degrading treatment, among others. The achievement of sexual health is thus closely associated with the protection of human rights.

Over the past three decades there has been a rapid expansion of the application of human rights to sexuality and sexual health matters, particularly relating to protection from discrimination and violence, and protection of freedom of expression and association, privacy and other rights, for women, men, transgender and intersex people, adolescents and other population groups. This has resulted in the production of an important body of human rights standards promoting sexual health and human rights. States have made legal and political commitments to protect the health of people, including their sexual health, through the application of human rights principles, expressed through national laws and policies and their implementation, recognizing that human rights principles have a strong role to play in promoting and protecting sexual health.

Spurred by public health evidence, scientific and social progress, as well as a growing body of international standards, working definitions of sexual health and sexuality have been developed *(4)* (see Box 1).

Box 1: Working definitions

- **Sexual health** is a state of physical, emotional, mental and social well-being in relation to sexuality; it is not merely the absence of disease, dysfunction or infirmity. Sexual health requires a positive and respectful approach to sexuality and sexual relationships, as well as the possibility of having pleasurable and safe sexual experiences, free of coercion, discrimination and violence. For sexual health to be attained and maintained, the sexual rights of all persons must be respected, protected and fulfilled.

- **Sexuality** is a central aspect of being human throughout life; it encompasses sex, gender identities and roles, sexual orientation, eroticism, pleasure, intimacy and reproduction. Sexuality is experienced and expressed in thoughts, fantasies, desires, beliefs, attitudes, values, behaviours, practices, roles and relationships. While sexuality can include all of these dimensions, not all of them are always experienced or expressed. Sexuality is influenced by the interaction of biological, psychological, social, economic, political, cultural, legal, historical, religious and spiritual factors.

1.2 Laws, human rights and their importance for sexual health

Human rights are codified in international and regional treaties, often also called conventions, covenants and charters, and are also incorporated at the national level in constitutions and laws. National constitutions, laws and highest court decisions thus provide national recognition of the human rights standards that are elaborated in these international and regional human rights treaties, which states ratify. Importantly, national laws often provide guarantees and legal frameworks for the elaboration of sexual-health-related policies, programmes and services, but sometimes they also impose limitations, and they thus have an impact on sexual health, both positive and negative. For example, laws that foster the dissemination of objective and comprehensive information and education on sexuality enable people to understand what protects or damages their sexual health, as well as to know where and how to seek further information, counselling and treatment if necessary. On the other hand, laws that restrict people's access to health services – for example, by requiring third-party authorization for services or by criminalizing certain consensual sexual behaviour – have the effect of excluding people from the health information and services they need.

Laws can also play an important role in ensuring accountability – a key human rights principle – at many levels, including, among others, establishing transparent monitoring and review processes to record health outcomes across a sexually diverse population, or the impact of various health interventions. Such review processes can help identify laws that have harmful effects and/or that contradict human rights. Laws can also establish guarantees for access to justice, redress and reparations mechanisms for people whose human rights are violated, which is central to accountability. States must also ensure that people are protected against human rights violations by non-state actors. An example of this would be a health insurance company that excludes certain people from being covered by insurance, purely on grounds of characteristics such as religious affiliation, gender, sexual orientation or health status.

Laws and regulations are pertinent to another key human rights principle: that of participation. It has been recognized that participation of affected populations in all stages of decision-making and implementation of policies and programmes is a precondition of sustainable development, and indeed, evidence shows that there is an association between participation of affected populations and health outcomes. In reality, many affected populations are unable to participate in assessing and making laws and regulations because of ongoing discrimination, often associated with increased exposure to violence and disease. For example, some states legally restrict transgender, lesbian, gay or sex-worker identified groups from registering as associations; others enact laws criminalizing their speech. All of these measures affect their ability to work against violence, HIV/AIDS and other issues of great importance to sexual health. At both the international and regional level, courts and human rights bodies have found these kinds of restrictive laws to be violations of fundamental rights of speech, association and protection from non-discrimination; in these decisions the basic principle of ensuring rights to participation in society are affirmed.

1.3 Legal and policy implications

The respect, protection and fulfilment of human rights, and the assurance of the highest attainable standard of sexual health, require states to bring their laws, as well as regulations, policies and practices, into line with international, regional and national human rights standards *(5)*.

In order to point the way to specific considerations for action that Member States can undertake, each chapter of this document includes a section on Legal and policy implications. The questions follow the framework of each chapter and they address: (i) whether national laws give recognition to the health and human rights topic in question; (ii) whether the particular topic or topics contained in the chapter are addressed through law; and (iii) overarching issues raised in the chapter. All the questions are based on a health and human rights rationale and the notion of state accountability.

For people working in public health and concerned about sexual health in particular, it is essential to understand the impact of certain laws on health broadly and on sexual health in particular, and to understand how human rights standards can be used to ensure supportive laws and thus improve health.

As a contribution to WHO's constitutional mandate to integrate human rights into its work, this report seeks to demonstrate the inextricable links among different dimensions of sexual health, human rights and the law, and in doing so, to help governments and health policy-makers improve sexual health through bringing their laws and policies into alignment with their own constitutional and international human rights obligations. Sexual health is an often neglected dimension of the continuum of care in the domain of reproductive, maternal, newborn, child and adolescent health. This report is offered as one important tool in the fulfilment of the fifth aspect of the WHO global reproductive health strategy adopted by the World Health Assembly in 2004: promoting sexual health *(5)*.

II. Methodology and limitations

This report is the result of extensive research and consultation globally over a period of seven years.

Starting from WHO's working definitions of sexual health and sexuality (see Chapter 1, Box 1), and recognizing that laws and policies can affect health as well as human rights, as outlined in the WHO global reproductive health strategy (5), the project's aim was to articulate the relevant international, regional and national human rights norms and standards that promote sexual health, and provide examples of national laws and jurisprudence that uphold these standards, together with evidence to support them.

Three important considerations drove the development of the project: (a) application of existing human rights standards as established by international, regional and national authoritative bodies; (b) national laws and jurisprudence are valid indicators of human rights standards, and they set the framework for operational actions; and (c) laws and their implementation have an impact on health.

2.1 Process

WHO convened a consultation in Geneva in February 2008, inviting various public health, legal and human rights experts to elaborate the scope, design and content of the project.

Nine human rights experts from the six WHO regions, and two experts with international and North American legal expertise (see Acknowledgements), were engaged to conduct research on laws and jurisprudence related to sexuality and sexual health at the international and regional levels and in selected countries, and to analyse and write up international/regional reports of the findings (6–13).

In May 2009, a meeting was held with the legal researchers to further develop the research strategy, including identifying the topical scope, research terms, sources of information, and inclusion/exclusion criteria for the legal and jurisprudential research. An analysis meeting was held in Berkeley, California, in January 2010, to examine international, regional and national findings and to set parameters to ensure consistency across the regional research reports in order to facilitate cross-regional analysis.

In parallel to the legal research, literature reviews of public health evidence were conducted to assess the documented impact of laws and their enforcement and implementation on sexual health and well-being in each of the eight identified topic areas (see section 2.2).

Upon completion of the legal and public health reviews, a small meeting of experts was held in Geneva in June 2011 to elaborate the methodology for the cross-regional analyses and the final outline and content of the report.

Between June 2011 and August 2012, a draft report was produced by a small expert group and presented to a larger expert group meeting in September 2012, at WHO in Geneva, for peer review. Participants were invited based on their diverse regional and multidisciplinary expertise. The report was then extensively revised based on feedback received from the meeting participants as well as from external reviewers.

2.2 Scope

The expert consultation in 2008 defined eight topic areas to reflect a holistic approach to sexual health, and to capture how laws address these issues and also how human rights standards elaborated in authoritative international, regional and legal documents relate to them.

The topics were chosen with regard to the following key criteria:

- demonstrated association with sexuality, sexual health and well-being;
- relevance to the fifth pillar of the WHO global reproductive health strategy – promoting sexual health – and to other WHO work in the area of sexual health;
- prioritization of poor and underserved populations and groups;
- intersection of human rights standards with the content of laws and their association with sexual health.

The eight topics identified were:

i.   **Non-discrimination,** including (non) discrimination based on sex, including issues related to: sexual harassment; age (special attention to adolescents); sexual orientation; gender identity and expression; marital status; health and other relevant status such as being a migrant or a prisoner.

ii. **Penalization of sexuality/sexual activities,** including: the (de)criminalization of same-sex sexual activity; (de)criminalization of (intentional) transmission of HIV; age of consent/statutory rape; and sexual activity in prisons and other state custodial institutions.

iii. **State regulation of marriage and family,** including: the (de)criminalization of sex outside marriage; consent to marriage; conditions placed on permission to marry, such as virginity testing and testing for HIV/STIs.

iv. **Gender identity/expression,** including: civil status registration; (de)criminalization of certain aspects of gender expression; access to health services; (non)discrimination and protection from violence.

v.   **Violence,** including domestic/intimate partner violence; sexual violence (including rape and in different contexts such as marriage or incarceration); female genital mutilation; police brutality/failure to respond due to sexuality or gender-related appearance/behaviour; hate crimes; honour crimes; and sexual exploitation, including trafficking of minors.

vi. **Availability, accessibility, acceptability and quality of sexual health services,** including: services for abortion, contraception, STI prevention, testing and treatment, and other relevant health services; and access to appropriate services for specific populations such as prisoners, refugees, injecting drug users, adolescents, the military, physically and mentally disabled people, trafficked people, and older people.

vii. **Information, education and expression related to sexuality and sexual health,** including: sexuality education; sexuality and sexual health information; erotic expression; and (de)criminalization of obscenity/indecency.

viii. **Sex work,** including: (de)criminalization; legalization/regulation; and (non) discrimination in access to health care and other services.

2.3 Search strategy and data sources

2.3.1 Human rights, legal and jurisprudential data

Three levels of document sources were culled and reviewed: international, regional and national. Regions were defined according to the WHO regions: African Region, Region of the Americas, Eastern Mediterranean Region, European Region, South-East Asian Region and the Western Pacific Region.

For each region, the researchers from each region made an in-depth review of both the regional human rights law and the laws and jurisprudence of selected countries, culling examples of national laws and highest court decisions according to the inclusion/exclusion criteria listed below. Based on grey literature and interviews with experts, they identified relevant national laws, which they then located and, where necessary, translated.

Sources of information

(a) *International sources:* United Nations (UN) human rights treaties; international humanitarian law (primarily the Geneva Conventions and their protocols); international criminal law (primarily the International Criminal Court's Rome Statute *[14]*, definitions of crimes, ad hoc and hybrid tribunal statutes and case law, and the UN Protocol to Prevent, Suppress and Punish Trafficking in Persons [Palermo Protocol; *15])*; refugee law (primarily the 1951 Convention relating to the Status of Refugees and its 1967 Protocol, and the authoritative *Handbook and guidelines on procedures and criteria for determining refugee status [16])*; international labour law (primarily the International Labour Organization [ILO] treaties); international political consensus documents; UN Human Rights Council resolutions; and UN treaty monitoring bodies' general comments/recommendations and decisions (see Table 1).[1]

(b) *Regional sources:* regional legally binding human rights treaties; other relevant regional legally binding treaties; relevant jurisprudence of regional human rights courts and other authoritative bodies; secondary legal sources (though not necessarily legally binding), such as regional resolutions and declarations, provided by relevant regional authoritative bodies.

(c) *National sources:* constitutions; national laws, such as civil codes, criminal codes, family laws, administrative laws if relevant, health-care laws, laws on HIV, and other laws relevant to sexual health and sexuality.

Inclusion criteria for human rights standards, laws and jurisprudence

1. close connection to sexuality and sexual health;

2. explicit reference to the sexual health needs of vulnerable/marginalized populations;

3. reflection of the respect, protection and fulfilment of human rights, expressed either explicitly in the law and/or reflected in particular provisions;

4. at the national level: state laws and highest court decisions only;

5. in federal legal systems: federal laws and state-level laws;

6. diverse national examples in the region;

7. identifiable primary sources of the text of laws and court decisions.

Exclusion criteria for human rights standards, laws and jurisprudence

• policies and lower-level regulations, unless they had a particular significance for understanding the content of a higher-level law;

• customary and religious laws;

---

1 Note: Reports of UN Special Rapporteurs were not systematically searched and analysed, but some of the most relevant reports are referenced in the text.

• draft and pending laws;

• implementation measures, unless explicitly articulated in laws and jurisprudence.

2.3.2 Public health data

Six reviews of the public health literature were conducted, to elucidate the possible association (or lack of association) between particular laws or policies and different sexual health conditions or outcomes. These six reviews covered: information, education and expression related to sex and sexuality; criminalization of consensual sexual behaviour; sex work; gender identity and expression; marriage; and sexual violence.

Sources of information

Multiple databases, including PubMed, Web of Science, Popline and Embase, were searched for primary sources of data, including epidemiological studies and reports by NGOs and other international or national institutions. Grey literature was reviewed in order to identify themes and primary sources, but papers identified in the grey literature were not included as data sources. Identified papers were summarized in a literature review for each of the six topics, including a list of keywords.

Inclusion criteria

• studies published from 1995 to 2011;

• specific reference to the particular topic area (e.g. sexuality education);

• reporting original findings with clear and valid methodologies;

• studies relying on secondary data, unclear methods, small sample sizes, etc., were only included if there were no other data on the subject area (clearly marked as less reliable sources);

• review articles and systematic reviews were only included in cases where access to original articles was impossible or the literature was too vast to review in detail;

• systematic reviews were included to provide an overall indication of the relationship between the topic area and sexual health.

Exclusion criteria

- opinion papers;

- papers describing intervention programmes without rigorous evaluation of health impact.

2.4 Critical assessment and synthesis of retrieved information

The January 2010 meeting (see section 2.1: Process) set the parameters for the critical assessment and analysis of the source materials.

Human rights standards: The international and regional human rights standards relating to the eight identified sexual health topic areas were established as the benchmark against which national laws and jurisprudence were assessed.

Legal and jurisprudential data: The legal and jurisprudential information retrieved was assessed as to whether it was (i) consonant with authoritative international and regional human rights standards, and (ii) relevant to sexual health.

Public health data: The public health information was assessed on the basis of the extent to which legal measures – for example the decriminalization of sex work – were associated with positive or negative health outcomes related to sexuality and well-being. Given that laws and their implementation do not readily lend themselves to epidemiological measurement, associations were assessed based on available studies that examined these outcomes as rigorously as possible.

For each sexual health topic area (see section 2.2: Scope) the following analytical framework was set:

- description of the topic from the health and well-being point of view;

- identification of relevant international and regional human rights standards for the topic;

- documented impact (positive and negative) of laws relating to sexual health and well-being;

- identification of legal and jurisprudential examples from different regions/countries of laws that demonstrate, either explicitly or implicitly, the protection of human rights and the sexual health and well-being of the population.

The following rules were followed in synthesizing the information retrieved:

- Issues for which clear examples, human rights standards and/or public health relevance were not identifiable were excluded from the report.

- The selection of national examples did not aim to provide a comprehensive review and analysis of all countries in the region.

- Identification of national laws did not indicate the existence of implementation measures.

- Laws that were identified throughout the legal assessment (based on our inclusion/exclusion criteria) were not analysed within their national, cultural, societal or political contexts; only the strict text of the laws was used.

- The protection of health needs of vulnerable/marginalized populations and human rights standards specifically established for their protection were systematically integrated across the report.

- Specific attention was paid to the health and human rights protections of adolescents.

The in-depth research into international, regional and selected national laws and human rights jurisprudence relating to sexuality and sexual health revealed an extensive number of laws, in a wide variety of countries, that deal in some way with sexuality and sexual health.

Many of the laws analysed demonstrated negative dimensions: they were clearly associated either with negative health outcomes (e.g. the penalization of adultery through flogging or even the death penalty) or with violations of human rights (e.g. the exclusion of unmarried people from receiving information and services related to contraception) or, most frequently, both.

In all regions of the world, however, examples were identified of laws and jurisprudence that both uphold human rights standards and aim to contribute to the promotion and protection of sexual health. The report particularly focuses on providing illustrative examples of laws and jurisprudential materials from different parts of the world that have a demonstrated positive effect on sexual health and that adhere to international, regional and/or national human rights norms and standards.

2.5 Peer review and document preparation

As mentioned in section 2.1 (Process), the first full report was subjected to extensive peer review at an international expert group meeting in September 2012, and subsequently by additional external expert reviewers from different disciplines.

Based on the analysis of relevant laws and court decisions against the key criteria listed under section 2.2 (Scope), selected results from the research were grouped under three main chapter headings, reflecting the ways in which aspects of sexual health are closely linked to human rights and the law

> Chapter 3: Health services for the promotion and protection of sexual health
>
> Chapter 4: Information and education for sexual health
>
> Chapter 5: Sexual and sexuality-related violence.

Issues related to discrimination, the health and human rights of vulnerable/marginalized populations and particular legal measures, such as the application of criminal law to consensual sexual behaviour, were integrated across these three chapters.

2.6 Limitations of the research and the report

The laws highlighted as examples of adherence to human rights standards and likely to promote sexual health represent a selection from each region under each topic. Thus, the mention of a law in one particular country is not an indication that there are no other such examples in other countries. It should also be borne in mind that laws are complex and many of the laws identified through the regional and international research and highlighted as positive may also contain negative aspects.

This report focuses on international human rights and common law as employed at the national level, but it is important to note that religious and customary laws and related legal mechanisms also play a central role in issues related to sexuality and sexual health. While these fall outside the scope of this report, there is a critical need for evidence to be generated around these and other systems of justice dispensation, and other community-based actors that influence the sexual health and well-being of local populations. The use of religious authority figures within the community to enforce compliance with social and religious standards of behaviour also needs to be documented in order to better protect the vulnerable.

The intersections of sexual health, human rights and the law are complex and certainly require much more than one report to articulate, analyse and understand. This analysis chose as a first step to focus on the letter of the law and the legal framework; the analysis focuses solely on the formal content of statutes, judicial decisions or other duly enacted laws. While human rights are codified in national laws, the respect, protection and fulfilment of human rights can only be fully achieved through the proper implementation of laws. This report, however, does not deal with implementation of laws, as such an undertaking requires a different methodology and should be the focus of a subsequent report. In a few places, reference is made to policies and programmes (i.e. evidence of implementation of the law), mostly to make explicit a particular point concerning a particular kind of law. The reader should therefore bear in mind that the report rests on the assumption that law can promote rights and enhance freedom, autonomy, and the health and well-being of individuals, but that it also acknowledges the limitations of the law alone as a tool for achieving development goals. This report should be read as a contribution to the discussion on how sexual health and human rights can be enhanced and protected, but not as a formula for their instant realization.

This report provides as a unique and innovative piece of research and analysis. Other UN organizations are examining the links between health, human rights and the law: the United Nations Development Programme's (UNDP's) Global Commission on HIV and the Law published its report in 2012 (17), and the Office of the High Commissioner for Human Rights (OHCHR) and United Nations Special Rapporteurs regularly report to the Human Rights Council on the impact of laws and policies on various aspects of sexual health. Nevertheless, this is the first report that combines these aspects, specifically with a public health emphasis.

Table 1: Core international human rights treaties and their optional protocols (and date of entry into force) relevant to the protection of human rights in the context of sexual and reproductive health

Treaty (date of adoption)	Monitoring body
International Covenant on Economic, Social and Cultural Rights (ICESCR) (1966)	**Committee on Economic, Social and Cultural Rights**
Optional Protocol to the International Covenant on Economic, Social and Cultural Rights (2008)	Committee on Economic, Social and Cultural Rights
International Covenant on Civil and Political Rights (ICCPR) (1966)	**Human Rights Committee[2]**
Optional Protocol to the International Covenant on Civil and Political Rights (1966)	Human Rights Committee
Second Optional Protocol to the International Covenant on Civil and Political Rights, aiming at the abolition of the death penalty (1989)	**Human Rights Committee**
International Convention on the Elimination of All Forms of Racial Discrimination (ICERD) (1965)	Committee on the Elimination of Racial Discrimination
Convention on the Elimination of All Forms of Discrimination Against Women (CEDAW) (1979)	**Committee on the Elimination of Discrimination Against Women**
Optional Protocol to the Convention on the Elimination of All Forms of Discrimination Against Women (1999)	Committee on the Elimination of Discrimination Against Women
Convention against Torture and Other Cruel, Inhuman or Degrading Treatment or Punishment (CAT) (1984)	**Committee Against Torture**
Optional Protocol to the Convention Against Torture and Other Cruel, Inhuman or Degrading Treatment or Punishment (2002)	UN Subcommittee on Prevention of Torture and other Cruel, Inhuman or Degrading Treatment or Punishment
Convention on the Rights of the Child (CRC) (1989)	**Committee on the Rights of the Child**
Optional Protocol to the Convention on the Rights of the Child on the sale of children, child prostitution and child pornography (2000)	Committee on the Rights of the Child
Optional Protocol to the Convention on the Rights of the Child on the involvement of children in armed conflict (2000)	
International Convention on the Protection of the Rights of all Migrant Workers and Members of their Families (ICRMW) (1990)	**Committee on Migrant Workers**
Convention on the Rights of Persons with Disabilities (CRPD) (2006)	**Committee on the Rights of Persons with Disabilities**
Optional Protocol to the Convention on the Rights of Persons with Disabilities (2006)	Committee on the Rights of Persons with Disabilities

---

2   The Human Rights Committee is sometimes also referred to as the Committee on Civil and Political Rights.

III. Health services for the promotion and protection of sexual health

3.1 Introduction

Ill health related to sexuality represents a significant disease burden throughout the world. This includes: morbidity and mortality related to HIV (18) and other STIs (19); morbidity and mortality linked to lack of access to contraception and safe abortion services (20); erectile dysfunction; the sequelae of sexual violence and female genital mutilation; and sexual and reproductive cancers (1).[3]

For example, sexually transmitted infections (STIs) are a significant cause of acute illness, infertility, long-term disability and death, with serious medical and psychological consequences for millions of men, women and adolescents. For people aged 15–49 years, an estimated 448 million new cases of four curable STIs (chlamydia, gonorrhoea, syphilis and trichomoniasis) occurred in 2005 (19), and these numbers are not diminishing. An estimated 35 million people in 2013 were living with HIV, a largely sexually transmitted infection (18), and while the incidence of HIV continues to fall, this is still a huge burden related to sexual health. Globally, the proportion of women living with HIV has remained stable at 50% of all those living with HIV, although women are more affected in sub-Saharan Africa and the Caribbean (18). Since the beginning of the HIV epidemic in the 1980s, men who have sex with men and transgender people have been disproportionately affected by HIV. The few existing epidemiological studies among transgender people have shown disproportionately high HIV prevalence, ranging from 8% to 68% depending on the context and the type of study carried out (21).

The continuing increase in the use of contraception since the 1960s (22) has contributed to a reduction in maternal mortality, and it is estimated that one in three deaths related to pregnancy and childbirth could be avoided if all women had access to contraceptive services (23). The increased use of modern contraceptive methods could not have been possible without the provision of services, whether public or private, through dedicated services or primary health care. Evidence shows that for adolescents, increased access to modern contraception, and particularly emergency contraception, protects them from negative health outcomes, and does not lead to unwanted sexual intercourse, unprotected intercourse, decreases in condom use, increased STIs or increased pregnancy rates (24–26). It has been estimated that a doubling of the current global investments in contraceptive and fertility regulation services – so that more women have better access to needed services – would reduce unintended pregnancies by more than two thirds, from 75 million to 22 million. But it would also reduce unsafe abortions by almost three quarters, from 20 million to 5.5 million, and deaths from unsafe abortion by more than four fifths, from 46 000 to 8000 (20). Thus, the provision of sexual and reproductive health services enables women to exercise control over their bodies in the case of unwanted pregnancies and helps to preserve their health.

Being able to be screened, counselled, diagnosed and treated appropriately for aspects of sexual health such as erectile dysfunction, the sequelae of sexual violence, female genital mutilation, reproductive tract infections that are not sexually transmitted, and sexual and reproductive cancers, is also critical for the protection and promotion of sexual health, as is having access to information and counselling related to sexuality (1). In addition, other health conditions such as cardiovascular disease, diabetes and cancer, all have a detrimental effect on the sexual and reproductive health of both men and women. For example, testicular cancer can threaten a young man's sexual and reproductive future, and prostate cancer can affect a man's mid- and later-life chances for a sexual life. Sexual dysfunction resulting from such conditions can be ameliorated through different approaches, usually requiring an interaction with the

---

[3] Some of the dimensions of sexual health overlap with what is classically included under reproductive health. Contraception and abortion in particular are frequently counted as part of reproductive health. They are included in this report on sexual health precisely because they are about NOT reproducing, but they are directly connected to sexuality and sexual activity.

health service *(27)*. Finally, for people whose deeply felt gender does not correspond to their sex assigned at birth, access to hormonal treatment or gender reassignment surgery, or other treatment, may be needed for the protection of their health including their sexual health.

Thus, the kinds of health services needed to promote and protect sexual health include: sexual health education and prevention information; sexuality counselling; identification and referral for victims of sexual violence and female genital mutilation; voluntary counselling, testing, treatment and follow-up for STIs, including HIV; screening, diagnosis, treatment and follow-up for reproductive tract infections, cancers and associated infertility; diagnosis and referral for sexual dysfunction and associated problems related to sexuality and intimate relationships; and safe abortion and post-abortion care. Such services may be integrated as part of primary health care or provided as stand-alone services, to address the most significant sexual health problems and concerns of the particular country, district or region *(1)*.

The respect, protection and fulfilment of internationally recognized human rights, such as the right to the highest attainable standard of health and the right to non-discrimination, require that all people have access to high quality and affordable health services, including those related to sexuality and sexual health, without discrimination *(28–36)*. The right to the highest attainable standard of health has been defined and elaborated as encompassing a variety of facilities, goods and services that must be available, accessible, acceptable and of good quality *(28, 29)*. It also includes the underlying determinants of health such as: access to safe and potable water and adequate sanitation; an adequate supply of safe food, nutrition and housing; healthy occupational and environmental conditions; as well as access to health-related education and information, including on sexual and reproductive health *(29, 37)*. Many national constitutions, such as those of the Republic of South Africa *(38)* and Portugal *(39)*, for example, explicitly guarantee the right to the highest attainable standard of health and specific aspects of it.

3.2 Creating enabling legal and regulatory frameworks and eliminating barriers to services for sexual health

The WHO global reproductive health strategy emphasizes that creating supportive legislative and regulatory frameworks and removing unnecessary restrictions from policies and regulations is likely to contribute significantly to improved access to services. To do this, states need to review and, if necessary, modify laws and policies to ensure that they facilitate universal and equitable access to reproductive and sexual health education, information and services *(5)*.

In a number of countries, many laws and regulations, or the lack of proper regulations, still present barriers to people accessing sexual health services. International human rights standards require that states not only refrain from activities that interfere with individuals' pursuit of their own health needs, but also remove legal and regulatory barriers to access to sexual and reproductive health services, such as laws or regulations that limit access to contraceptives *(28, 29, 40)*. States must also ensure that both state-supported (public) and private health services are regulated and monitored for adherence to health and human rights standards *(29, 41, 42)*.

Barriers to sexual health that are susceptible to regulation by law include: access to essential medicines, conscientious objection by health-care providers, availability and quality of health-care providers and facilities, and criminalization of certain services.

3.2.1 Access to essential medicines

Essential medicines are those that satisfy the priority health care needs of the population. They are selected based on public health relevance and evidence on efficacy, safety and comparative cost-effectiveness *(43)*. Access to essential medicines is guaranteed as part of the right to health; they must be available within the context of functioning health systems at all times, in adequate amounts, in the appropriate forms and dosages, with assured quality and at a price the individual and the community can afford *(29, 44, 45)*. Yet medicines needed for the promotion of sexual health, such as antiretrovirals for HIV, emergency contraception, or mifepristone and misoprostol for medical abortion – all of which are included on the WHO Model List of Essential Medicines *(46)* – are often either not available (due to intellectual property laws) or are restricted or prohibited by law. This situation has been challenged in various countries, including Colombia *(47)*, Mexico *(48)*, Peru *(49)*, and England and Wales *(50)*, resulting in the overturning of such restrictions or prohibitions. Some countries have declared contraception a "public good" and provide subsidized or free services for this aspect of sexual health (e.g. Canada; *51, 52*).

3.2.2 Conscientious objection by health-care providers

Another major barrier to sexual health services in some countries is the refusal by some health-care providers to provide sexual and reproductive health services on grounds of conscientious objection. By claiming conscientious objection, health-care professionals or institutions exempt themselves from providing or participating in the provision of certain services on religious, moral or philosophical grounds. This has affected a wide range of procedures and treatments, including abortion and post-abortion care, components of assisted reproductive technologies relating to embryo manipulation or selection, contraceptive services including emergency contraception, treatment in cases of unavoidable pregnancy loss or maternal illness during pregnancy, and prenatal diagnosis *(53)*. While most health-care providers who claim conscientious objection are obstetricians and gynaecologists, such objections have also come from pharmacists, nurses, anaesthesiologists and cleaning staff. Some public health institutions have informally refused to provide certain reproductive health services based on the beliefs of individual hospital administrators *(54)*.

While other regulatory and health system barriers also hinder women's right to obtain abortion services, conscientious objection is unique because of the tension existing between protecting, respecting and fulfilling a woman's rights, and a health-care provider's

own right to follow his or her moral conscience *(55)*. This situation leads to people's health being put in jeopardy when they are denied the services they need *(53, 55)*.

International human rights standards clearly stipulate that, although the right to freedom of thought, conscience and religion is protected by international human rights law, freedom to manifest one's religion or beliefs may be subject to limitations in order to protect the fundamental human rights of others *(32)*. Specifically, human rights and health system standards stipulate that health services should be organized in such a way as to ensure that an effective exercise of the freedom of conscience of health-care professionals does not prevent people, with special attention to women, from obtaining access to services to which they are entitled under the applicable legislation *(56–60)*. Therefore, laws and regulations should not allow health-care providers or institutions to impede people's access to legal health services *(28, 61–63)*. Health-care professionals who claim conscientious objection must refer people to a willing and trained service provider in the same or another easily accessible health-care facility. Where such referral is not possible, the health-care professional who objects must provide safe services to save an individual's life or to prevent damage to her health *(59, 60)*.

Some human rights bodies have explicitly addressed conscientious objection in the context of contraceptive service provision, stating that where women can only obtain contraceptives from a pharmacy, pharmacists cannot give precedence to their own religious beliefs and impose them on others as justification for their refusal to sell such products *(64)*. States have particular responsibility to ensure that adolescents are not deprived of any sexual and reproductive health information or services due to providers' conscientious objection *(40)*.

3.2.3 Availability and quality of health-care facilities and providers

The availability of health-care facilities and trained providers within reach of the entire population is essential to ensuring access to sexual health services. Some national laws stipulate that only doctors can perform certain services. In the area of sexual health, many services do not necessarily have to be provided by a physician, but can be competently provided by nurses, midwives or auxiliary nurses *(65, 66)*. Particularly in places where there are few qualified doctors, this kind of "task shifting" renders services more accessible *(67)*, increasing access to and use of contraception, for example *(68–71)*. International human rights standards, while emphasizing the importance of appropriately trained health-care providers with up-to-date skills and knowledge, do not specify the degree of qualification, leaving this for individual countries to regulate as appropriate. Some national laws, such as in South Africa *(72)*, specifically make provision for different levels of providers.

The right to the highest attainable standard of health, including sexual health, places an obligation on governments to ensure that health-care facilities, goods and services are of good quality *(29)*. In addition to the guarantee of confidentiality, privacy and informed consent (see sections 3.3.1 and 3.3.2), this requires that services have "skilled medical personnel, scientifically approved and unexpired drugs and hospital equipment, safe and potable water, and adequate sanitation" *(29)*.

3.2.4. Criminalization of sexual-health-related services

Laws that prohibit or criminalize the use of certain medical procedures represent, by definition, a barrier to access. Such laws and other legal restrictions may prevent access to certain commodities needed for sexual and reproductive health (e.g. contraceptives), they may directly outlaw a particular service (e.g. abortion), or they may ban the provision of sexual and reproductive information through school-based or other education programmes. In practice, these laws affect a wide range of individuals *(73, 74)*. Criminal law is also used to punish HIV transmission and a wide range of consensual sexual conduct occurring between competent persons (see section 3.4).

These legal restrictions on sexual and reproductive health services are likely to have serious implications for health *(74)*. Restricting legal access to abortion, for example, does not decrease the need for

abortion, but it is likely to increase the number of women seeking illegal and unsafe abortions, leading to increased morbidity and mortality. Legal restrictions also lead many women to seek services in other states or countries *(75, 76)*, which is costly, delays access and creates social inequities *(59)*.

International and regional human rights bodies and national courts have increasingly called for the removal of all barriers interfering with access to sexual and reproductive health information and services, including the criminalization of access to and provision of such information and services *(29, 31, 40, 74, 77)*. They call for the reform of laws that interfere with the equal enjoyment of rights by women *(78)*, including those laws that criminalize and restrict medical procedures needed only by women and that punish women who undergo these procedures *(79)*.

3.3 Ensuring quality and respect of human rights in the provision of sexual health services

The way in which services are provided has long been recognized as a crucial determinant of whether, and to what extent, people seek health services when needed. Studies have shown that adherence to quality of care standards results in outcomes such as women's satisfaction with services and an increase in contraceptive use *(80–83)*. Factors that are key to quality include: a guarantee of privacy and confidentiality; fostering informed decision-making; skilled health-care providers; and quality supplies and equipment.

Human rights bodies have also called on states to ensure timely and affordable access to good quality health services, including for adolescents, delivered in a way that ensures informed consent, respects dignity, guarantees confidentiality, and is sensitive to people's needs and perspectives *(28, 31, 37, 40)*.

3.3.1 Guarantee of privacy and confidentiality

Sexual health encompasses issues related to sexuality, sexual practices, contraception and sexually transmitted infections (STIs), which are perceived as sensitive in many settings. Many people may be reluctant to discuss them or reveal relevant information. At the same time, health workers are often entrusted with this private information by their patients, such that respect for confidentiality and privacy is essential. If individuals fear that confidentiality and privacy are not guaranteed in the health-care environment, they may avoid seeking services, thus putting their health in jeopardy (28, 84–88).

The right to privacy means that individuals should not be subject to arbitrary or unlawful interference with their privacy and should enjoy protection of the law in this respect (89). Many constitutions, national laws and regulations guarantee the right to privacy and confidentiality. However, in practice this may not be applied to the provision of sexual health services (59, 60, 85, 90). In line with human rights commitments, and in order to promote the health and development of all, states are encouraged to strictly respect the right to privacy and confidentiality, including with regard to advice, counselling and services related to sexual health. Health-care providers have an obligation to keep medical information confidential – both written records and verbal communications. Such information may only be disclosed with the consent of the patient (28, 29, 40, 59, 60, 65, 84, 91).

3.3.2 Fostering informed decision-making

Because many of the decisions relating to sexual health may have an impact on people's ability to have a safe and satisfying sexual life and to have or not have children, informed decision-making – which includes informed refusal of certain interventions or medicines – is particularly important. Individuals have the right to be fully informed about any treatment, intervention or other health services they may seek or undergo. In the area of sexual health, informed decision-making includes fully understanding and accepting (or declining) a particular service, such as a diagnostic test for an STI or HIV, or intervention, such as sterilization or abortion (92). Informed decision-making invokes several elements of human rights that are indivisible, interdependent and interrelated. In addition to the right to health, these include the right to self-determination including reproductive

self-determination, freedom from discrimination, security and dignity of the human person, and freedom of thought and expression (93). In order to make a free and fully informed decision, the individual concerned must have adequate reasoning faculties and be in possession of all relevant facts at the time consent is given (59, 60, 93).

People should not be pressured, forced, coerced or in any other way persuaded to undergo treatment or interventions against their will. Certain populations, such as people with disabilities, indigenous and minority people, women living with HIV, sex workers, drug users, and transgender and intersex people, may be particularly vulnerable to coercion or to being persuaded to undergo certain procedures, such as intrauterine device (IUD) insertion or sterilization, without their free and fully informed choice and consent (91). Children in particular may be subjected to certain procedures that have an impact on their future sexuality and sexual health, such as children with intersex conditions receiving medically unnecessary, so-called sex normalizing surgery before they are old enough to participate in the decision (91), and young girls undergoing genital mutilation (94) (see also Chapter 5). States have an obligation to protect these individuals from coercion and discrimination (29) and to ensure that rights to autonomy, bodily integrity and dignity, as well as the principle of acting in the child's best interests, are protected (40).

The right to informed decision-making, including the requirement for informed consent, may be recognized in national laws and is often covered in medical ethical codes, but many states' laws or policies fail to explicitly recognize it. Nonetheless, states have the legal duty to ensure that services are provided in a way that presents information in a clear and understandable way, including the likely benefits and potential adverse effects of proposed procedures and available alternatives (28), so that clients can make a choice. Censoring, withholding or intentionally misrepresenting information about sexual and reproductive health services can result in a lack of access to services or delays, which, in the case of abortion services for example, increase health risks for women (59). International and regional human rights standards have affirmed the requirement for full information in relation to interventions, including for sexual health *(28, 56, 92)*.

3.3.3 Skilled health-care personnel

Health-care providers who are inadequately trained are not able to provide appropriate health services. In the field of sexual health, specific training is needed, especially in the area of counselling related to sexuality, and more generally for dealing with many different kinds of clients with a non-judgemental and respectful attitude, with sensitivity to gender and human rights dimensions *(1, 65)*. For example, health personnel who have to assist with childbirth for a woman who has been infibulated (a form of genital mutilation whereby the inner and/ or outer lips of the vulva are cut and then stitched together, narrowing the vaginal orifice) require specific training, not only to help in the delivery of the baby and ensuring the woman's health, but also in counselling and follow-up with the woman in a way that is both culturally appropriate and aligned with medical ethics and human rights *(95–97)*. Untrained health-care providers may be unable or unwilling to provide appropriate health care for transgender people *(98)*. Health workers may wrongly assume that people with disabilities are asexual, or that people with intellectual disabilities cannot become parents. All such inappropriate training or gaps in training are likely to be associated with poor health outcomes *(99)*.

In line with human rights standards, states must ensure that the training of doctors and other health and medical personnel meets appropriate standards of education, skill and ethical codes of conduct *(29)*. These assurances are often made through laws and regulations at the national level. WHO guidance on core competencies for sexual and reproductive health emphasizes that all workers at the primary health care level dealing with sexual and reproductive health must be adequately trained, prepared and supported in their work, and this must be accompanied by a supportive infrastructure and supervision system to ensure that these health workers maintain an adequate level of competence *(65)*. This is especially important in remote and rural areas where the knowledge, skills and attitudes of health workers may be life-saving, while a lack of competence could be life-threatening *(65)*.

3.3.4 Quality of supplies and equipment

Due in part to the high cost of many medicines needed for sexual health care (see section 3.2.1), the widespread availability of cheaper but sub-standard medicines poses a serious health risk to many people *(100)*. Ranging from inactive or ineffective preparations to mixtures of harmful toxic substances, sub-standard products have been found among, for example, contraceptive pills *(101)* and antibiotics in different parts of the world *(102)*.

Outmoded or old equipment may also pose a health risk, when safer and more effective equipment exists at competitive prices. For example, in a number of countries physicians still use dilatation and curettage (D&C) to perform abortion even though vacuum aspiration (either manual or electric) has been shown to be effective, less painful, and easier to perform, requiring fewer accompanying procedures (e.g. general anaesthesia) and less hospital equipment (e.g. operating theatres) *(59)*.

3.4 Elimination of discrimination in access to health services – addressing the specific needs of particular populations

Inequity and inequalities in access to health care around the world are well documented *(103)*. Very often, such inequities are related to socioeconomic factors, including income and place of residence (rural or urban), but they may also be related to characteristics such as living with a disability. The provision of services related to sexuality and sexual health presents additional difficulties related to societal perceptions (also held by health-care providers) of acceptable sexual behaviour, which are often heightened by the fact that laws, policies and practices may exclude certain categories of people from health services.

Laws which preclude anyone's access to needed health services, including those for all dimensions of sexual health, violate human rights and are likely to be associated with ill health which might have been prevented *(28, 29, 40)*. By contrast, a legal and policy framework that ensures access to needed services, even for marginalized groups, is likely to result in positive health outcomes. As just one example, the provision of sexual health services and information to female sex workers has been shown to lead to increased condom use and reduction in HIV and STI prevalence *(104, 105)*, a finding that has been consistent across African and Asian settings *(106)*. International human rights standards make it clear that the grounds on which discrimination is prohibited are non-exhaustive, and include age, sex, disability, marital and family status, sexual orientation, gender identity and health status (e.g. HIV), all of which are closely associated with sexual health, and that equal treatment is essential for specific population groups (i.e. regardless of race, colour, language, religion, political or other opinion, national or social origin, property, place of residence, economic and social situation), as part of their right to access sexual and reproductive health services without discrimination *(40, 107, 108)*. For example, persons with disabilities should be provided with the same range, quality and standard of free or affordable health care and programmes as other people, including in the area of sexual and reproductive health *(36)*.

The right to non-discrimination is often enshrined in national constitutions. Some states have elaborated specific laws on non-discrimination, and some include specific provisions for non-discrimination in other laws. These standards, however, are not always translated into policies and regulations.

Some specific examples of continued legal barriers, health and human rights standards, as well as good practice in law, are given below, relating to adolescents, people who experience discrimination based on their marital status, incarcerated people, migrants and asylum seekers, people living with HIV, people living with disabilities, lesbian, gay, transgender, gender variant and intersex people, and people engaged in sex work.

3.4.1 Adolescents (under 18 years of age)[4]

An adolescent's decision to go to a health service for sexual health care or advice is likely to be influenced by whether or not they will get into trouble with parents or guardians, or even with the law, in places where sexual activity under a certain age or by unmarried people is against the law. In many cultures, social norms strongly forbid premarital sex, such that unmarried adolescents are likely to be wary about seeking care even if they have a painful genital ulcer or a possible unwanted pregnancy. This problematic situation is compounded by the fact that in many countries adolescents under 18 are not recognized under the law as competent to consent to treatment on their own.

In order to respect and protect human rights, states must ensure that health systems and services are able to meet the specific sexual and reproductive health needs of adolescents, including contraception and safe abortion services *(40)*. States are required to ensure that comprehensive sexual and reproductive health services are available and accessible to both married and unmarried adolescents without discrimination of any kind and with special consideration to underserved areas and populations *(31, 40, 84)*. States also need to ensure that adolescents are not deprived of any sexual and reproductive health information or services due to providers' conscientious objection (see section 3.2.2) *(40)*.

Human rights standards at the international, regional and national levels are well developed regarding the protection of adolescents under 18 from discrimination in accessing both information and services for sexual health. They also require states

---

4 The World Health Organization defines adolescents as people aged 10–19, and this definition is widely reflected in health statistics for the age ranges 10–14 and 15–19, although not all relevant health statistics use these age ranges. From a legal point of view, adolescents below the age of 18 (minors) are recognized as holders of all human rights, specifically enshrined in the Convention on the Rights of the Child, and elaborated in General Comment No. 4 on Adolescent health and development in the context of the Convention on the Rights of the Child (31). Adolescents below the age of 18 are entitled to special protection measures and, according to their evolving capacities, they can progressively exercise their rights.

to guarantee adolescents' rights to privacy and confidentiality by providing sexual and reproductive health services without parental consent on the basis of their evolving capacities (31, 40, 84). At the same time parents require adequate education and information that enhances their capacity to build relationships of trust and confidence with their adolescent children, so that issues of sexuality and sexual behaviour can be openly discussed and the adolescents' rights respected (40). Several national laws reflect international and regional human rights standards that apply to adolescents, including being entitled to confidentiality when obtaining condoms, contraceptives or contraceptive advice (e.g. South Africa; 109).

3.4.2 Marital status

Access to sexual and reproductive health services may be dependent on a person's marital status and whether and how marriage is regulated in a given country. There are various aspects of marriage regulations that can affect access to health care and related issues, such as access to medical records, health insurance and social benefits.

A number of countries still have laws and policies that prohibit health-care providers from delivering contraceptive services or other sexual and reproductive health services to unmarried women seeking such services. This barrier to needed services contributes to the burden of ill health faced by many unmarried women (59, 60). Moreover, the requirement that women clients be married may be accompanied by a requirement for the husband to authorize his wife's access to contraceptives or abortion services. International human rights standards specify that States Parties should not restrict women's access to health services or clinics that provide these services on the grounds that women do not have the authorization of husbands, partners, parents or health authorities, or because they are unmarried (28, 110).

In settings where extramarital or premarital sexual behaviour is criminalized, people who engage in such conduct are at risk of stigma, discrimination, violence and arrest, and they may avoid or be unable to access needed health services (such as

contraceptives, STI treatment or safe, legal abortion services), with detrimental effects on their health (23, 111). This is particularly the case for women, since the sanctions and penalties are, in some places, significantly more serious for women than for men – or even if the penalties are the same they are more likely to be enforced to punish women than to punish men (112).

Even in cases where adultery is not itself a criminal offence, societal disapproval may still lead to legal and social consequences for women, such as denying them custody of their children or inheritance of property through divorce cases. In some parts of the world it may lead to social ostracism (e.g. Sri Lanka; 112, 113).

International human right bodies have urged countries to eliminate laws that classify adultery as a criminal offence, noting that such laws give rise to punishments ranging from fines to flogging and death by stoning or hanging. They have particularly condemned laws that sentence women to death for adulterous activities as evidence of discrimination. They have also raised concerns about the serious discriminatory effects of penal laws that provide for either mitigation of sentence, or exculpation of guilt of persons who wound or kill women presumed to be adulterous (79, 112, 114). In addition, United Nations guidelines encourage states to consider granting refugee status, including specific asylum protections, to women and girls fleeing severe penalties for transgressing conventional social mores, which may include sanctions for sex outside of marriage (115).

In a number of countries across the regions of Africa, South-East Asia and the Western Pacific, laws criminalizing adultery and fornication still exist and are applied to varying degrees. Many other countries, however, have decriminalized sex outside of marriage (e.g. Argentina and Brazil; 116, 117), and high courts have adopted judicial decisions to decriminalize adultery. The argumentation of the Constitutional Court of Guatemala in 1996, for example, included the fact that the regulation of adultery by the Criminal Code was a form of sex discrimination and therefore was in violation of the Constitution (118).

Another dimension of marital status that may hinder access to health services is the lack of legal recognition for marriages or civil partnerships for same-sex couples on an equal basis with heterosexual couples. This may result in denying access to health services and health-related benefits, since in many countries marriage is the basis for entitlement to a wide range of social rights and benefits.

International and regional human rights bodies increasingly recognize the protection of individuals from discrimination on the basis of sexual orientation and gender identity, to ensure that unmarried same-sex couples are treated in the same way and entitled to the same benefits as unmarried heterosexual couples (13, 119–121). An increasing number of countries have instituted legal reforms making domestic partnerships or civil unions more equal to marriage in terms of benefits and social protection (122). A number of national courts have stated in their decisions that non-discrimination is a fundamental aspect of personhood and that the right to non-discrimination and equality imply that cohabiting same-sex partners should be able to partake of the status, entitlements and responsibilities accorded by law to cohabiting, opposite-sex couples (e.g. Brazil, Israel, New Zealand, Slovenia; 123–127).

Various countries around the world have legalized same-sex marriages to protect fundamental human rights, including access to health services and social benefits (e.g. Argentina, Canada, France, the Netherlands, New Zealand, South Africa; 128–133).

3.4.3 Incarceration

Being compulsorily confined to one location, people in prison and other detention facilities are reliant upon the incarcerating authority for access to health services. Sexual activities take place in correctional facilities. Few studies have examined the public health impact of access to sexual health services in correctional settings, but it has been found that high levels of discrimination against those living with HIV motivate prisoners to hide their HIV status (134) and that those with a history of incarceration within 12 months of initiating highly-active antiretroviral treatment (HAART) are more likely not to adhere to treatment. On the other hand, the widespread

availability of HAART in the prison system in the United States of America (USA), for example, has resulted in a decrease in AIDS mortality in prisons, with the rate declining from 1010 deaths per 100 000 in 1995 to 12 deaths per 100 000 in 2006 (135, 136). With regard to contraception, available evidence suggests that providing female inmates access to contraception while incarcerated results in increased use following release (137).

International human rights standards consistently stress that prisoners must have access to preventative and remedial health services and that their conditions of detention and punishment must not be prejudicial to their health (138–143). They also include clauses stating that the rules must be applied without discrimination on the grounds of sex (138, 140–143) or "other status" (138, 140–142).

3.4.4 Migrants and asylum seekers

Undocumented migrants are particularly vulnerable to violations of their rights to sexual health services due to their illegal status, lack of health insurance and/or practical difficulties in accessing care. The fear of being subjected to deportation may impede undocumented migrants from seeking treatment. By the very nature of living illegally, and possibly also due to language barriers, undocumented migrants are likely to find it difficult to access information about services and treatment (see also Chapter 5).

International human rights standards hold that the enjoyment of human rights, including access to health care, should not be limited to citizens of states but should be available to all individuals, regardless of nationality or whether or not they are stateless, such as asylum seekers, refugees, migrant workers and other persons, who may find themselves in the territory or subject to the jurisdiction of the state (144). Some national laws guarantee emergency care regardless of a person's legal status (e.g. UK; 145), and international policy guidelines strongly support efforts to scale up voluntary testing and counselling services and unequivocally oppose mandatory or compulsory testing for HIV (146).

3.4.5 HIV status

Although being HIV-positive is not itself indicative of sexual transmission of the infection, individuals are often discriminated against for their HIV-positive status based on a presumption of sexual activity that is often considered socially unacceptable. In addition, in response to the fact that most HIV infections are due to sexual transmission (147), a number of countries criminalized transmission of, or exposure to, HIV (17), fuelling stigma, discrimination and fear, and discouraging people from getting tested for HIV (148–150), thus undermining public health interventions to address the epidemic.

Even where persons living with HIV/AIDS may be able, in principle, to access health services and information in the same way as others, fear of discrimination, stigma and violence may prevent them from doing so. Discrimination against people living with HIV is widespread, and is associated with higher levels of stress, depression, suicidal ideation, low self-esteem and poorer quality of life (151), as well as a lower likelihood of seeking HIV services and a higher likelihood of reporting poor access to care (152–154).

HIV transmission has been criminalized in various ways. In some countries criminal laws have been applied through a specific provision in the criminal code and/or a provision that allows for a charge of rape to be escalated to "aggravated rape" if the victim is thought to have been infected with HIV as a result. In some cases, HIV transmission is included under generic crimes related to public health, which punish the propagation of disease or epidemics, and/or the infliction of "personal injury" or "grievous bodily harm" (155).[5]

Contrary to the HIV-prevention rationale that such laws will act as a deterrent and provide retribution, there is no evidence to show that broad application

of the criminal law to HIV transmission achieves either criminal justice or public health goals (150, 159). On the contrary, such laws fuel stigma, discrimination and fear, discouraging people from being tested to find out their HIV status (148–150), and undermining public health interventions to address the epidemic (160). Thus, such laws may actually increase rather decrease HIV transmission (17, 73, 161).

Women are particularly affected by these laws since they often learn that they are HIV-positive before their male partners do, since they are more likely to access health services (150, 162). Furthermore, for many women it is either difficult or impossible to negotiate safer sex or to disclose their status to a partner for fear of violence, abandonment or other negative consequences (150, 163, 164), and they may therefore face prosecution as a result of their failure to disclose their status. Criminal laws have also been used against women who transmit HIV to their infants if they have not taken the necessary steps to prevent transmission. Such use of criminal law has been strongly condemned by human rights bodies (17).

Various human rights and political bodies have expressed concern about the harmful effects of broadly criminalizing the transmission of HIV (17, 73, 150, 165, 166). International policy guidance recommends against specific criminalization of HIV transmission (150). Human rights bodies as well as United Nations' specialized agencies, such as UNAIDS, have stated that the criminalization of HIV transmission in the instance of intentional, malicious transmission is the only circumstance in which the use of criminal law may be appropriate in relation to HIV (73, 150). States are urged to limit criminalization to those rare cases of intentional transmission, where a person knows his or her HIV-positive status, acts with the intent to transmit HIV, and does in fact transmit it.

Human rights bodies have called on states to ensure that a person's actual or perceived health status, including HIV status, is not a barrier to realizing human rights. When HIV status is used as the basis for differential treatment with regard to access to health care, education, employment, travel, social security, housing and asylum, this amounts

---

[5]   Questions of whether an HIV-infected person who knows his or her status has told his or her sexual partner(s) or not, whether the intercourse was protected or not, whether the accused had a specific intention to infect the partner and whether the non-infected partner became infected, have been, and still are, the subject of intense debate in courts around the world, with widely varying positions (156–158).

to restricting human rights and it constitutes discrimination *(107)*. International human rights standards affirm that the right to non-discrimination includes protection of children living with HIV and people with presumed same-sex conduct *(84)*. Human rights standards also disallow the restriction of movement or incarceration of people with transmissible diseases (e.g. HIV/AIDS) on grounds of national security or the preservation of public order, unless such serious measures can be justified *(29)*.

To protect the human rights of people living with HIV, states have been called on to implement laws that help to ensure that persons living with HIV/AIDS can access health services, including antiretroviral therapy *(35)*. This might mean, as in the case of the Philippines, for example, explicitly prohibiting hospitals and health institutions from denying a person with HIV/AIDS access to health services or charging them more for those services than a person without HIV/AIDS *(167)*.

International guidance also suggests that such laws should be consistent with states' international human rights obligations *(150, 168)* and that instead of applying criminal law to HIV transmission, governments should expand programmes that have been proven to reduce HIV transmission while protecting the human rights both of people living with HIV and those who are HIV-negative *(150)*.

3.4.6 Disability

People with disabilities have been found to face multiple barriers in access to health services. A world health survey found that people with disabilities were twice as likely to find health-care provider skills and equipment inadequate to meet their needs, three times as likely to be denied care, and four times as likely to be treated badly as non-disabled people. They were also 50% more likely to experience catastrophic health expenditure. Health-care providers may consider that people with intellectual disabilities or other disabilities should not have a sexual life, reproduce or look after children, and therefore should not need sexual and reproductive health services. Furthermore, health-care settings may be physically inaccessible and health information may be unavailable in different formats *(99)*.

International human rights standards state that people with disabilities are entitled to health services, including those for sexual and reproductive health, on an equal basis with others, and to have control over their fertility *(36, 169)*. In particular, sexual health information and education should be made available in accessible formats. People with disabilities are entitled to the support and time they require to make informed decisions about matters of sexual and reproductive health *(36)*. People with disabilities should not be subject to involuntary and/ or forced interventions such as sterilization *(36, 91)*.

3.4.7 Sexual orientation and gender identity

Many people in the world are stigmatized and discriminated against because of their actual or perceived sexual orientation or gender identity. Among other disparities, lesbian, gay and transgender people are significantly more likely than the general population to be targeted for violence and harassment, to contract HIV, and to be at risk for mental health concerns such as depression and suicide *(73, 74, 121, 170)* (see also Chapter 5).

In settings where same-sex consensual sexual behaviour is against the law, people may be deterred from seeking health services out of fear of being arrested and prosecuted *(73, 74, 121, 170)*.

Even in countries where it is not deemed a criminal offence to be gay, when they use health services, people perceived as being lesbian, gay and transgender are often discriminated against and ill treated by medical providers, reducing the likelihood that they will seek services in the future. Refusal to make clinic appointments, refusal to treat, or treatment with gross disrespect, violation of medical privacy, private shaming and public disparagement are among the discriminatory practices and abuses that have been reported, along with hurried and inferior care *(121, 153, 171)*. Such attitudes from health-care providers make many people reluctant to share personal and medical information, jeopardizing their overall health and their access to health services including those for sexual health *(21, 172–174)*. Gay, lesbian, transgender and intersex people (see also sections 3.4.8 and 3.4.9) are often coerced and forced to undergo certain procedures, such as forced sterilization, forced abortion and/ or forced anal examination *(21, 175–177)* (see also Chapter 5).

The right of everyone to the enjoyment of the highest attainable standard of health includes entitlements to available and accessible health-care facilities for all people without discrimination on any grounds, including gender identity and sexual orientation *(28, 29, 84)*. It also includes freedoms such as the right to have control over one's own body, and to be free from non-consensual medical treatment, experimentation and torture *(178)*. United Nations human rights treaty monitoring bodies emphasize both dimensions and recognize sexual orientation and gender identity as prohibited grounds for discrimination in achieving the highest attainable standard of health *(40, 107, 179)*. International, regional and national human rights standards, and a growing body of health standards that respect and protect human rights, provide clear benchmarks on how the health and human rights of gay, lesbian, transgender, gender variant and intersex people should be respected, protected and fulfilled *(40, 107, 179–185)*. Laws can play an important role in providing safeguards and guarantees in this regard *(121)*.

International human rights standards explicitly call for the decriminalization of consensual same-sex sexual activity, and have established that such criminal laws are in breach of human rights *(28, 77, 179–181, 186–193)*. The consequences to health and well-being of the criminalization of same-sex sexual activity have been spelt out in global and national decisions and recommendations, including the recognition that criminal law has no public health value *(17, 108, 194)*.

There are many countries of the world that have either never criminalized homosexuality, sodomy or consensual same-sex sexual activity, or have decriminalized them *(17, 121)*. For example, Colombia decriminalized consensual same-sex sexual activity in 1980 *(195)*, Chile did so in 1998 *(196)*, Nicaragua in 2008 *(197)*, and Fiji in 2009 *(198)*. South Africa is among those countries that explicitly protect the right to non-discrimination on the grounds of sexual orientation *(194, 199)*.

3.4.8 Transgender and gender variant people[6]

Transgender and gender variant people worldwide experience substantial health disparities and barriers in accessing appropriate health services. Due to perceived gender-nonconformity, in nearly all societies these people are stigmatized and discriminated against, and often experience high levels of violence from police, gangs, family members, health-care providers and others. Stigmatization, discrimination, and legal, economic and social marginalization and exclusion impede their access to necessities such as appropriate and good quality health care, social welfare, housing, education and employment. Some forms of gender expression are criminalized in many countries, and transgender and gender variant people are often subjected to compulsory medical interventions without an opportunity for informed decision-making and choice. All these factors affect their overall health and well-being, including sexual health. In addition, not being able to live according to one's self-identified gender is likely to be a source of distress, exacerbating other forms of ill health *(73, 200, 201)*.

When transgender and gender variant people seek health services, they are often rejected or mistreated by health-care providers, and as a result,

---

[6] This report uses the terms "transgender" and "gender variant" to refer to people who identify themselves with a different sex/gender from that assigned to them at birth, while recognizing that, among various terms used globally, the term "trans" is gaining in recognition and popularity. Around the world there have always been people whose gender identity and expression differ from cultural expectations associated with the sex/gender they were assigned at birth. Across cultures, regions and societies, people may identify as transsexual, transgender, transvestites, travestis and cross-dressers, among others. Various cultural and indigenous terms are also used to describe a wide and diverse range of gender identities, including: *hijra* and *aravani* (India), *meti* (Nepal), *fa'afafine* (Samoa, America Samoa, Tokelau), *transpinay* (Philippines), *meme* (Namibia), *muxe* (Mexico), *omeggid* (Panama). Someone born male who identifies as female may use the term "male-to-female", (MtF), "transwoman", "transgender woman", "transfeminine", or simply "woman" to describe her gender identity. Someone born female who identifies as male may use the term "female-to-male" (FtM), "transman", "transgender man", "transmasculine", or simply "man" to describe his identity.

transgender and gender variant people may avoid going to health services at all (202, 203). Services are particularly inaccessible for those who are poor (204–209).

Besides requiring access to health services that other people also need (including primary care, gynaecological, obstetric, urological and HIV care), transgender and gender variant people may also need access to specific kinds of health services, although services and care related to gender transition are only desired by some. Some people make this transition socially through a change of name, dress or other aspects of gender expression, without any medical procedures (98, 201, 210, 211). Services related to gender transition may include hormonal therapies, surgical procedures, psychological counselling, permanent hair removal and/or voice therapy. Depending on individual needs, transgender and gender variant people may need different transition-related services at different times in their lives (98).

Evidence shows that in many cases, acquiring physical sex characteristics congruent with experienced gender identity (such as by undergoing gender-affirming surgery) improves health, well-being and quality of life, including better self-esteem and improved physical, mental, emotional and social functioning (206, 212–219), and some have shown improvement in sexual function and satisfaction (218, 220).

Many transgender and gender variant people have to travel long distances to find clinics that can provide appropriate, comprehensive care. Although the number is increasing, there are still very few non-discriminatory, appropriate health services available and accessible to transgender and gender variant people, which are non-pathologizing, supportive and confidential, and which prioritize an individual's informed decision-making. Health professionals often lack technical competence as, internationally, there are very few medical curricula, health standards and professional training programmes that have incorporated a comprehensive approach to transgender health care (98, 201, 208, 210, 211, 221–223).

Withholding or denying access to information and to quality transition-related services may have multiple health-related ramifications, including anxiety, depression, substance abuse and suicidal thoughts or behaviour (98, 224–226). Where health services are expensive and not subsidized, or are disrespectful, transgender and gender variant people may obtain hormones of dubious quality from outside the health system, often through the black market or the Internet, and take them without proper supervision of dosage (208, 227–234). The improper use of sex hormones can lead to serious health problems such as liver damage, blood clotting, deep vein thrombosis, hypertension and potentially harmful impacts on pubertal growth (214, 235, 236). If care from a trained person is not available, transgender people may also end up receiving crude methods of castration by unqualified people, with serious risks such as urinary stricture, septic infection and even death (208, 237, 238). Transgender women may choose to inject free-floating silicone, or other harmful substances such as cooking oil, as a faster and more accessible way to achieve the body they desire (206).

An additional problem is that recognition of the need for transition-related health services does not always translate into funding for such care; private and public insurers often do not offer, or may specifically exclude, coverage for medical procedures for gender transition, and there are substantial variations in which services are covered under what conditions (239–241).

Human rights standards call for the availability, accessibility, acceptability and quality of health information, including for transgender and gender variant people, and require that all those seeking services should be treated with respect and dignity, free from discrimination (29, 40, 107, 242). Some regional standards specifically call for the consideration of the specific needs of transgender persons in the development of national health plans, including suicide prevention measures, health surveys, medical curricula, training courses and materials, and when monitoring and evaluating the quality of health services (175). Furthermore, access to, and reimbursement of, gender-affirming surgery has been specifically addressed by international and regional human rights and professional bodies *(121, 175, 243, 244)*.

An increasing number of countries have revised or are revising laws and regulations relating to accessing transition-related services. In Argentina, for example, the 2012 Law includes provisions for coverage of all medical costs related to procedures and treatment for transgender people based on their informed decision-making without additional requirements *(245)*.

Furthermore, legal gender recognition has an impact on people's ability to live in accordance with their self-identified gender, including being able to change their name and legal gender if they so wish. Identification is required for many activities in life, from accessing health services and applying for housing, to travelling across borders and applying for employment or education *(121, 175, 201, 246)*.

Human rights bodies recognize that obstructing legal determination of gender identity and imposing arbitrary requirements, such as sterilization, is contradictory to human rights, including the right to privacy and the right of transgender people to personal development and to physical and moral security *(121, 175, 178, 247, 248)*. They urge states to recognize the right of transgender persons to change their legal gender by permitting the issuance of new birth certificates *(249–251)*.

Some countries only allow legal change of gender identity if certain requirements are met, such as a mental health diagnosis, unmarried status (or divorce) and body modifications, which often include surgical procedures, hormonal therapies, and chemical or surgical sterilization *(121, 175, 201)*. In several parts of the world, such requirements have been found to be a violation of human rights, and have been successfully challenged by national human rights and legislative bodies (e.g. Austria, Germany, Italy and New Zealand; *252–256)*. Increasingly, countries are adopting laws without any such requirements (e.g. Argentina, Denmark and Malta; *245, 257, 258)*.

Some transgender and gender variant people do not identify as male or female, but as a third gender.

Recognizing such phenomena, legal recognition of a third gender has been implemented in a number of countries throughout the world (e.g. Nepal and Pakistan; *201, 259–261)*.

3.4.9 Intersex people[7]

Intersex people may face discrimination and stigma in the health system, in many cases being subjected to lack of quality of care, institutional violence and forced interventions throughout their lifetime *(178, 262, 263)*.

A major concern for intersex people is that so-called sex normalizing procedures are often undertaken during their infancy and childhood, to alter their bodies, particularly the sexual organs, to make them conform to gendered physical norms, including through repeated surgeries, hormonal interventions and other measures. As a result, such children may be subjected to medically unnecessary, often irreversible, interventions that may have lifelong consequences for their physical and mental health, including irreversible termination of all or some of their reproductive and sexual capacity. Medical procedures may sometimes be justified in cases of conditions that pose a health risk or are considered life-threatening. Such procedures, however, are sometimes proposed on the basis of weak evidence, without discussing and considering alternative solutions *(178, 262, 264–270)*.

Increasingly, concerns are being raised by intersex people, their caregivers, medical professionals and human rights bodies that these interventions often take place without the informed consent of the children involved and/or without even seeking the informed consent of their parents *(178, 262, 264, 270–273)*. Parents often consent to medical intervention for their children in circumstances where full information is lacking and without any discussion of alternatives *(263, 274)*.

According to human rights standards, intersex persons should be able to access health services on the same basis as others, free from coercion,

---

[7] The health and human rights concerns faced by intersex people may be similar to those faced by transgender people, and in other respects their concerns may be different. See also section 3.4.8.

discrimination and violence *(29, 107, 242)*. Human rights bodies and ethical and health professional organizations have recommended that free and informed consent should be ensured in medical interventions for people with intersex conditions, including full information, orally and in writing, on the suggested treatment, its justification and alternatives *(178, 264, 275)*.

These organizations have also recommended that medical and psychological professionals should be educated and trained about physical, biological and sexual diversity and integrity, and that they should properly inform patients and their parents of the consequences of surgical and other medical interventions and provide additional support *(91, 176, 264, 268, 271, 276)*. It has also been recommended that investigation should be undertaken into incidents of surgical and other medical treatment of intersex people without informed consent and that legal provisions should be adopted in order to provide remedies and redress to the victims of such treatment, including adequate compensation *(91, 264)*.

3.4.10 People engaged in sex work[8]

In many countries sex work and allied activities are criminalized or severely restricted. Criminalization and application of other punitive regulations to sex work foster discriminatory practices and stigmatizing social attitudes and drive sex work underground, making health services hard to reach *(73, 277–280)*.

Criminalization can take various forms. Some countries criminalize every act relating to exchanging sex for money, while in others the actual act of selling or buying sex is not a crime, but all surrounding acts are criminalized, such as

---

[8] This report uses the terms "sex work", "sex worker" and "people engaged in sex work" to refer to persons making an autonomous decision to be in sex work. It does not address those who are forced into sex work or those who are understood to be trafficked. This aspect is dealt with in Chapter 5. The term "sex work" is used in preference to "prostitution" or "commercial sex work". However, when references are made to specific laws or policies, the terminology of the law is used.

soliciting for the purpose of prostitution, renting a room for this purpose, or brothel-keeping *(17, 281, 282)*. In addition to actual criminal laws, a wide range of administrative and local or municipal laws related to "public order" are frequently applied to people engaged in sex work; they may be charged with offences such as vagrancy, public nuisance, stopping the flow of traffic, being in parks or other public places after hours, obscenity, public alcohol consumption and the like *(283)*.

Criminalization has a negative impact on sex workers' access to health services *(278, 284–286)*. Sex workers may assume that they will be denied services, or may fear arrest, prosecution and imprisonment if they go to services, including for diagnosis and treatment of STIs, including HIV *(278, 284–286)*. They may have more difficulty obtaining products such as male and female condoms, post-exposure prophylaxis following unprotected sex and rape, drug treatment and other harm reduction services *(280)*, as well as maternal health, contraceptive and abortion services *(170, 287)*.

Even if they reach services, sex workers are likely to face poor treatment. Research in countries as different as Canada, Nepal and South Africa describe sex workers as experiencing discrimination and stigmatization by health-care providers, including in clinics specifically designed for sex workers *(284, 288–290)*.

Some regulatory regimes impose mandatory health checks or health cards, meaning that people engaged in sex work must go for medical check-ups every so many weeks and if they are diagnosed with an STI, their card — which enables them to work legally – may be confiscated either temporarily or permanently (in the case of HIV). This situation can give police officers (whose role is to monitor sex worker compliance with health regulations) the power to force people engaged in sex work to undergo health checks and create opportunities for corruption, blackmailing and other serious abuses of police powers, including bribery, rape, and extended and arbitrary detention to extract fines *(290, 291)*.

International human rights bodies have called on states, at a minimum, to ensure: the rights of all sex workers, whether men, women or transgender people, to access sexual health services; that they are free from violence or discrimination, whether by state agents or private persons; and that they have access to equal protection of the law *(15, 28, 73, 292, 293)*.

International guidelines published in 2012 by WHO, entitled *Prevention and treatment of HIV and other sexually transmitted infections for sex workers in low- and middle-income countries*, recommend that all countries should work toward decriminalization of sex work and elimination of the unjust application of non-criminal laws and regulations against people engaged in sex work. Specifically, it is recommended that governments should establish anti-discrimination and other rights-respecting laws to protect against discrimination and violence, and other violations of rights faced by people engaged in sex work in order to realize their human rights and reduce their vulnerability to HIV infection and the impact of AIDS. The guidelines also recommend that anti-discrimination laws and regulations should guarantee sex workers' rights to social, health and financial services. Health services should be made available, accessible and acceptable to people engaged in sex work based on the principles of avoidance of stigma, non-discrimination and the right to health *(170)*.

A variety of measures have been put in place by states to safeguard the health and rights of sex workers. Some states have completely decriminalized sex work and elaborated regulations that cover health and safety issues, such as formulation and implementation of workplace occupational health and safety standards for the brothel environment, and provision of contraception services and sexual health information (e.g. Australia; *294, 295)*. The positive impact of such measures include, for example, increased condom use among brothel-based sex workers (up to 100% in some instances), significantly reduced prevalence rates of STIs, and very low rates of HIV infection *(294, 296, 297)*. It has been reported that decriminalization of prostitution has had a positive impact on sex

workers' access to health services and occupational health and safety programmes *(294)*.

Some countries or particular states/provinces in a country have decriminalized some or all forms of sex work and have legalized it by recognizing sex work as a form of labour and employment *(282)*. These legal regimes aim to give people engaged in sex work access to legal and other protections available to other workers, such as coverage by occupational health and safety legislation and access to health services and social and medical insurance (e.g. the Netherlands, New Zealand; *298, 299)*. Labour law has also been used to uphold the human rights of people engaged in sex work, including protection against illegal dismissal and guaranteeing maternity protection (e.g. Colombia and South Africa; *300, 301)*, and access to social security benefits (e.g. Colombia; *300)*.

Even in some countries with punitive laws and other regulations against selling or buying sex, there have been efforts to limit the harmful effects of these laws on the health, safety and rights of people engaged in sex work, including protection from forced eviction, police brutality and violence (e.g. Bangladesh; *302)*.

Criminalization of sex work can particularly impact access to health services for young people under 18 engaged in sex work. Even though international human rights law, international labour law and international criminal law consider any engagement of persons under 18 in sex work a crime *(15, 293, 303)*, millions of young people and children are engaged in the commercial sex sector. Many legal regimes that criminalize sex work simultaneously prosecute not only the people who coerce minors into sex work but also the minors themselves. Prosecution of people under 18 as criminal offenders achieves little other than stigmatizing young people and making their lives even more difficult. International human rights standards hold that states have an obligation "to enact and enforce laws to prohibit all forms of sexual exploitation and related trafficking; to collaborate with other States Parties to eliminate inter-country trafficking; and to provide appropriate health and counselling services to adolescents who have been sexually exploited, making sure that they are treated as victims and not as offenders" *(31)*. Strategies that offer education and alternative ways of making a living for people under 18 engaging in sex work are most likely to be productive *(304)*.

3.5 Conclusion

Ill health related to sexuality represents a significant disease burden throughout the world. Access to appropriate health services for sexual health is an essential part of addressing such ill health.

International, regional and national human rights standards make it clear that states must ensure, to the greatest extent possible, that everyone has access to essential health services, including those for sexual health. The state is responsible for ensuring the availability, accessibility, acceptability and quality of health services, in both the public and private sphere. This involves ensuring access through removing both direct and indirect legal and policy barriers such as: restrictions on essential medicines; providers' refusal to provide services; restrictions on health-care providers; criminalization of certain sexual health services and medical procedures; and requirements for third-party authorization. Access to quality care must also be guaranteed through appropriate training of health-care providers, through the safeguarding of privacy, confidentiality and informed decision-making, and by ensuring adequate supplies of good quality medicines and up-to-date equipment.

Excluding anyone from accessing needed health services results in preventable ill health. Those who may have difficulty accessing needed sexual health services include adolescents, people who are unmarried, those in detention, migrants and asylum seekers, people living with HIV, people living with disabilities, people with same-sex sexual orientation, transgender and intersex people, and people engaged in sex work. International human rights law prohibits any discrimination in access to health care and underlying determinants of health. Nearly all states enshrine the right to non-discrimination in their constitutions, and some states have elaborated specific laws on non-discrimination and/or have

included specific provisions for non-discrimination in other laws, including in relation to accessibility of health services. However, such standards are not always translated into policies and practices. States must provide legal guarantees for access to health care free from discrimination, and must implement them through policies and practices.

3.6 Legal and policy implications

On the basis of the human rights standards described in this chapter, and in order to safeguard sexual health and well-being, the following questions should be examined by those who are responsible for setting enabling legal and policy frameworks.

1. Do laws, regulations and/or policies guarantee the provision of comprehensive health services in relation to sexuality and sexual health?

2. Do national human rights standards and/or laws guarantee the following:

- access to essential medicines including those needed for sexual health and well-being?

- the exercise of conscientious objection does not jeopardize people's access to health services in relation to sexuality and sexual health?

- the provision of health services that are essential for safeguarding the highest attainable standard of sexual health?

- that categories of health-care providers who can provide certain services related to sexuality and sexual health are not restricted if appropriately trained providers can deliver services safely and efficiently?

- that people's rights to confidentiality and privacy are explicitly protected?

- that any consultation, treatment or intervention is done on the basis of the health service users' informed decision-making?

- that health-care personnel are educated and trained to be able to provide appropriate services related to sexuality and sexual health?

- availability of quality supplies and equipment necessary for the provision of services related to sexuality and sexual health?

3. Do national human rights standards and/or laws provide guarantees for the accessibility of health services without discrimination and take into account the rights and health care needs of specific population groups, including adolescents, people who are unmarried or cannot marry because of the law, those in prison and other detention facilities, migrants and asylum seekers, people living with HIV, people living with disabilities, people with same-sex sexual orientation, transgender, gender variant and intersex people, and people engaged in sex work?

4. Has the state considered the negative health (including sexual health) consequences of criminalization of the provision of sexual and reproductive health services, and the criminalization of consensual sexual activity, and has it taken all necessary measures to decriminalize such acts?

5. Does the state consider that establishing and applying specific criminal provisions on HIV transmission can be counter-productive for health and the respect, protection and fulfilment of human rights, and that general criminal law should be used strictly for intentional transmission of HIV?

6. Do laws and/or policies ensure participation of various stakeholders and affected populations with regard to the elaboration of laws, policies, programmes and services related to health services/ health information and education/violence?

IV. Information and education for sexual health

4.1 Introduction

Information and education, including comprehensive sexuality education, are crucial for sexual health in several respects. They provide people with the knowledge and opportunity to make informed choices about sexual matters, including whether or not to enter into, and pursue, a safe and pleasurable sexual life, as well as how to protect themselves against HIV, other sexually transmitted infections (STIs) and unwanted pregnancy. Sexuality education and information also help people to break silences about sexual violence, sexual exploitation or abuse, and inspire those who suffer from problems related to sex or sexuality to seek help.

4.2 Defining sexuality information and education

As used in this report, "sexuality information" refers to information pertinent to sexual health, including information about sex and sexuality, about different forms of relationships and sexual practices, as well as ideas and opinions which convey diverse perspectives on sexuality. It also includes medical, social and scientific information, such as information about sexual function and dysfunction, the effectiveness and side-effects of various contraceptive methods, and how to protect oneself against HIV and other STIs.

Comprehensive sexuality education is understood to include accurate, age-appropriate, scientifically supported information on sexual health and sexuality as an aspect of being human, but it also covers issues of non-discrimination and equality, tolerance, safety, and respect for the rights of others. Comprehensive sexuality education is aimed at building an understanding of the positive aspects of sexuality, as well as ways to prevent ill health and when and how to seek assistance for ill health, abuse or other sexuality-related concerns. Comprehensive sexuality education is delivered through trained teachers using age- and context-appropriate pedagogical methods. It is a critical component of

promoting health and well-being, and needs to be understood as part of a broader system that includes access to services (1, 305).

In some societies, traditions and rituals for transmitting information about sexuality to young people may no longer take place. In others, open discussions about sexuality between adults and young people, or even among young people, are strongly discouraged. In many communities, young people are exposed to several different – and often conflicting – sources of information and values about sexuality and gender, such as parents, teachers, peers and the media (increasingly the Internet). Parents are often reluctant to engage in discussion of sexual matters with children because of cultural norms, as well as their own lack of knowledge or discomfort (305). This is why the provision of accurate, evidence-based information and education about sexuality and sexual health is so important.

Evidence from a range of countries indicates that information about sexuality and sexual health imparted through comprehensive sexuality education can improve sexual health outcomes, including delayed sexual debut, fewer unintended pregnancies, and increased use of condoms or other forms of contraception (305–311). Sexuality education programmes can contribute to building a sense of agency and enabling people to express their ideas, emotions, values, questions and concerns (312). Programmes that are well designed and implemented can improve young people's health-related knowledge, attitudes and skills, and their access to health services (305, 313–315). These are essential for achieving the primary goal of sexuality education: to equip people with the knowledge, skills and values to make informed and responsible choices about their sexual lives (305).

Reviews of evidence about sexual health programmes affirm the importance of building skills and capacity rather than focusing only on knowledge transfer (310), since knowledge alone does not necessarily lead to behaviour change (308, 309). For example, interventions that combine education, skill-building and contraceptive promotion have been shown to lower the rate of unintended pregnancy (310), and education interventions that are complemented by sexual negotiation skills can increase condom use in the short term *(316)*. The duration and intensity of programmes as well as the use of trained facilitators are also important for success *(311)*. In particular, a rights-promoting approach to sexuality education requires the participation and contribution of young people, particularly adolescents *(1)*.

Within the broader community, well designed sexuality information and education programmes can have a positive effect on sexual health. For example, the community intervention Stepping Stones, in South Africa, uses participatory learning approaches to build knowledge and communication skills and to stimulate critical reflection with regard to gender roles, sexual health, HIV/AIDS and gender violence within the broader community context. The intervention showed sustained reduction in the incidence of herpes simplex virus type 2 in men and women, and in the incidence of male violence against women, although no impact on HIV in women was found *(317–319)*.

4.3 Legal restrictions on sexuality information and education

Laws can create an enabling environment for the promotion and protection of health, including sexual health, but they can also pose barriers to people accessing sexuality information and education. Because sexuality is considered to be a sensitive topic in many societies, sexuality-related information and education have often – historically and still today – been considered "obscene", been censored, and in some instances provision of such information has been or still is criminalized. Laws that impose such restrictions are likely to contribute to people being exposed to risks – sometimes life-threatening, such as STIs including HIV, unwanted pregnancies and unsafe abortion – that they might otherwise have been able to avoid *(59, 74)*.

A diverse array of national laws provide the framework for governing what is permissible in speech, publications, performance, research and other forms of expression, and what must be censored, all with implications for sexual health. These laws include criminal codes, intellectual

property law, and administrative laws. Limitations elaborated in criminal law often use terms such as "obscene", "indecent", "offensive", "pornographic", "prurient" or "against public morals" to indicate material that cannot be published, distributed, purchased or viewed/read. Frequently, such laws do not define what is covered by those terms, such that their interpretation is subjective and thus the application of the law may not be supportive of people's need for comprehensive sexual health information and education *(320)*.

4.4 Human rights standards and legal protections

The freedom to seek, receive and impart information and ideas of all kinds, regardless of frontiers, either orally, in writing or in print, in the form of art, or through any other media, is a fundamental human right that cannot be arbitrarily restricted *(89, 321–323)*. Human rights standards clearly articulate that states must proactively put in the public domain information of public interest, including information related to sexual health, and make every effort to ensure easy, prompt, effective and practical access to such information *(29, 40, 324)*. This includes the fact that people must have guaranteed access to sexuality education, including information about contraceptives, that enables them to decide freely and responsibly the number and spacing of their children, as well as access to specific educational information to help ensure the health and well-being of families *(37, 40, 110, 325, 326)*. States must also take legislative and other measures to combat harmful practices, such as female genital mutilation (FGM) and early/child marriage, including the creation of public awareness in all sectors of society regarding harmful practices *(37)*.

A growing number of governments around the world are confirming their commitment to providing sexuality information and education as a priority essential to achieving national goals for development, health and education. In 2006, African health ministers adopted a plan of action for realizing sexual and reproductive health and rights, with provision of sexuality education within and out of school as a key strategy *(327)*. Two years later, health and education ministers from across

Latin America and the Caribbean came together in Mexico City to sign a historic declaration affirming a mandate for national school-based sexuality and HIV education throughout the region. The declaration advocates for strengthening comprehensive sexuality education and for making it a core area of instruction in both primary and secondary schools in the region *(328)*.

Some states have promulgated laws that make specific provision for sexuality information and education, based on the right to education. In Portugal, for example, such a law came into operation in 1984 *(329)* and has since been complemented by several other laws and decrees, including a law which makes sexuality education compulsory in private and public primary, secondary and professional schools *(330)*.

International and regional human rights standards clearly stipulate that states must refrain from censoring, withholding or intentionally misrepresenting health-related information, including sexuality education and information *(29, 84, 323, 331)*. Provision of information is an essential part of good quality sexuality and reproductive health services. Any obstruction of this is an interference with the right to impart and receive information, and it can result in delays or lack of access to services, thus exposing people to greater health risks *(59, 60, 332)*.

In a number of countries of different regions, national laws relating to HIV/AIDS in particular have been put in place to specify the kind of information that is needed to protect sexual health, thus counteracting the tendency to censor information that might otherwise be deemed "obscene". Some of these laws aim to foster the promotion of awareness and education about HIV/AIDS and its sexual transmission as a central part of the strategy to combat the epidemic *(333, 334)*. Others call for the establishment of specific programming for vulnerable and high-risk groups, including for people in penitentiaries and prisons, mental health institutions and military institutions, as well as education for the general public through the mass media *(335)*. Some laws clearly specify that materials with sexuality-related content should not be considered harmful or pornographic when their purpose is the dissemination of scientific, artistic

or technical ideas, or education about sexuality, human reproductive function, and the prevention of STIs and adolescent pregnancy, provided that the materials have been approved by the competent authority *(336)*.

4.5 Ensuring no arbitrary or unnecessary restrictions to information and education related to sexuality and sexual health for people under 18

For most young people, sexual activity with partners begins between the ages of 15 and 19 years regardless of the law, and for some it is even younger *(337)*. People under 18 years of age therefore need information and education about sexuality and sexual health, to support them in protecting their physical and mental health and well-being.

International human rights standards call on states to provide access to comprehensive and scientifically accurate sexuality education as part of the respect, protection and fulfilment of all individuals' rights to education, health and information. This includes information on family planning and contraceptives, the dangers of early pregnancy, the prevention of HIV/AIDS and other STIs, and information aimed at addressing cultural and other taboos surrounding adolescent sexuality *(31, 34, 40, 84)*. States are also encouraged to ensure that adolescents are actively involved in the design and dissemination of information through a variety of channels beyond schools, including youth organizations, religious, community and other groups, and the media *(31)*.

Health services are an important source of information on sexual health. International and regional human rights standards make clear that, in accordance with their evolving capacities, children should have access to confidential counselling and advice without the consent of a parent or legal guardian, where this is assessed by the professionals working with the child to be in the child's best interests. States should review and consider allowing children to consent to certain medical treatments and services without the permission of a parent or guardian, such as HIV testing and sexual and reproductive health services, including education and guidance on sexual health, contraception and safe abortion *(40, 338, 339)*.

Acting in the best interests of the child is a key human rights standard governing the actions of both the state and parents/guardians, who also have responsibility for the education of their children *(34, 84)*. This standard implies that, while the parents or guardians may take steps to raise their children consistent with their religious and cultural beliefs, and may choose the form of primary education, yet the rights of the child to objective and scientifically supported information, commensurate with their evolving capacity, is coupled with the duty of the state to present information and education in an objective manner to that child, through formal as well as informal channels *(84)*. This set of rights and duties means that parents can share their values and perspectives with their children, but cannot bar their children from receiving scientifically accurate sexuality-related information and education *(31, 40, 84, 340)*. This may also mean that parents/guardians can send their children to a school of their choosing with religious or other approaches to education, but the schools themselves are subject to regulation by national law including in relation to the provision of compulsory sexuality education *(340)*.

The importance of providing objective and scientific information and education in schools was upheld by the Colombian Constitutional Court after a challenge was made to the education law, which makes age-appropriate sexuality education a compulsory course in the preschool, basic and middle levels of all public and private schools. The Court emphasized the necessity of comprehensive sexuality education, among other things, for counteracting misinformation from other sources about sexuality, which might be damaging to individuals *(341–346)*.

4.6 Conclusion

Access to information and education relating to sexuality and sexual health is essential for people to be able to protect their health and make informed decisions about their sexual and reproductive lives. Evidence shows that access to such information as well as to comprehensive sexuality education,

which not only provides information but also builds personal communication skills, is associated with positive health outcomes.

The importance of the state providing sexuality information and comprehensive sexuality education is reinforced by international human rights standards that place legally binding obligations on governments to take steps to ensure that both adults and adolescents have access to such information and education, as well as the obligation not to obstruct people from having such access.

While states and parents have a duty to protect children from harm, this must be balanced with the duty of the state to provide children with information and education essential for their lives, their sexual health and their well-being, commensurate with their evolving capacities.

4.7 Legal and policy implications

In order to safeguard the sexual health and well-being of all, and on the basis of the human rights standards described in this chapter, the following questions should be examined by those who are responsible for setting enabling legal and policy frameworks in each country.

1. Does the state specifically recognize the right to seek, receive and impart information regarding human sexuality and sexual health?

2. Do laws and policies ensure the ability of all people to access comprehensive and scientifically accurate information and education necessary for achieving and maintaining sexual health?

3. Does the state prohibit censorship and the withholding or intentional misrepresentation of scientifically accurate sexual-health-related information?

4. Are policies in place to provide rights-based, age-appropriate, scientifically accurate and comprehensive sexuality information and education to those under 18 years of age through different means?

5. Do laws and/or policies ensure participation of various stakeholders and affected populations with regard to the elaboration of laws, policies, programmes and services related to health services/health information and education/violence?

V. Sexual and sexuality-related violence

5.1 Introduction

Over the past three decades, extensive research in all regions of the world has brought to light the extent of sexual violence[9] and sexuality-related violence[10] (121, 347–349). Sexual violence has a profound impact on physical and mental health. As well as causing physical injury, it is associated with an increased risk of a range of sexual and reproductive health problems, with both immediate and long-term consequences (350). People living in violent relationships, for example, may be unable to make sexual and reproductive choices, either due to being directly subjected to forced or coerced sex, or because they are unable to control or negotiate the use of contraception and condoms (351, 352). This puts them at risk of unwanted pregnancy and unsafe abortion (for women), and sexually transmitted infections (STIs), including HIV (349, 353–355). Intimate partner violence in pregnancy increases the likelihood of abortion, miscarriage, stillbirth, preterm delivery and low birth weight (356). People subjected to violence, including sexual and sexuality-related violence, have been found to be at increased risk of depression, post-traumatic stress disorder, sleep difficulties, eating disorders and emotional distress (347, 351, 357).

Recent global prevalence figures indicate that, overall, 35% of women worldwide have experienced either intimate partner violence or non-partner sexual violence in their lifetime. On average, 30% of women who have been in a relationship report that they have experienced some form of physical or sexual violence by their partner. Globally, as many as 38% of murders of women are committed by an intimate partner (349). Data indicate that there is a higher incidence of sexual violence directed against women and girls (350). However, sexual violence and sexuality-related violence can be, and is, directed against anyone – women, men, girls, boys, transgender people and intersex people – and particularly against people in positions of vulnerability, such as people engaged in sex work, migrants, internally displaced persons and refugees, and people with disabilities. For example, increasing attention is being paid to sexual violence against men in conflict situations (360, 361). In the last decade, sexualized violence against men and boys – including rape, sexual torture, mutilation of the genitals, sexual humiliation, sexual enslavement, forced incest and forced rape – has been reported in 25 armed conflicts across the world (362).

Sexual and sexuality-related violence serve as a form of punishment and control, which may be committed by both non-state actors such as family members, neighbours or co-workers, as well as by agents of the state such as police, with the intention of inducing shame and diminishing the reputation of the victim of violence. These forms of violence stem from other forms of inequality, and serve to reinforce hierarchies of power based on gender, class, race, ethnicity, caste, sexual orientation, gender identity and expression, or other important social divisions (121, 358). Victims of sexual violence may perceive themselves to be responsible, or may actually be held responsible by others, for the violence. They feel shame, dishonour, humiliation, guilt and stigmatization, all of which contribute to making it difficult to report incidents of violence, as well as to seek treatment and care for related physical and psychological injuries, thus compounding the health problems. Sexual violence is thus responsible for a significant disease burden (359).

Violence, including sexual violence and sexuality-related violence, is a violation of fundamental human rights, most notably the rights to life, to be free from torture and inhuman and degrading treatment, to the highest attainable standard of health, and to bodily integrity, dignity and self-determination (29, 40, 78, 292,

---

9 Sexual violence is defined as: any act, attempt to obtain a sexual act, unwanted sexual comments or advances, or acts to traffic, or otherwise directed, against a person's sexuality using coercion, by any person regardless of their relationship to the victim, in any setting, including but not limited to home and work (348).

10 The term "sexuality-related violence" is used in this report to signify violence – sexual or not – that is committed against a person because of their sexual characteristics or behaviour, or violence which has an impact on a person's sexual health.

363). Addressing violence against women in particular, international and regional human rights standards have made clear that the elimination of violence against women is essential for women's individual and social development and their full and equal participation in all sectors and spheres of society. Human rights bodies have specifically condemned traditional attitudes that regard women as subordinate to men, particularly because they perpetuate practices involving violence or coercion, the effect of which is to deprive women of the enjoyment of many of their human rights *(292)*.

Under international and regional human rights law, states have a responsibility to protect all individuals from all forms of violence. In line with the human rights concept of "due diligence", which applies to all persons, states must adopt legislative, administrative, social and economic measures necessary to prevent, investigate and punish acts of violence including rape, sexual violence, homophobic violence, female genital mutilation and trafficking into forced prostitution, whether perpetrated by the state or by private persons *(37, 363, 364)*. States should also provide effective remedies, compensation and a mechanism for seeking redress *(41, 365, 366, 367)*.

Many states have adopted national legislation to address the issue of domestic and intimate partner violence, including sexual violence. Yet there are still national laws that do not recognize the diversity of forms or contexts of sexual violence, often leading to serious negative consequences for health and rights *(368)*. On the other hand, international and regional human rights standards now define the diversity of forms of violence, perpetrators and victims, and a growing number of national laws and jurisprudence reflect this, as highlighted in this chapter.

This chapter focuses on those forms of violence that are directly sexual or related to sexuality, including rape, child sexual abuse, forced marriage, trafficking into forced prostitution, regardless of the gender or sex of the victim. It also addresses other forms of violence affecting bodily and sexual integrity such as female genital mutilation, coercive practices within health services that directly affect people's sexual and reproductive health, and violence committed

against persons because of their real or perceived sexual practices, behaviour and expression, including hate crimes and so-called honour killings.

5.2 Health, human rights and legal implications of different forms of sexual and sexuality-related violence

5.2.1 Sexual assault including rape

Someone who is sexually assaulted, including someone who is raped or coerced into unwanted sexual intercourse, has little or no control over the situation, and the sexual health consequences are serious: possible unwanted pregnancy, and the need for abortion, which might be unsafe; exposure to STIs including HIV; and other reproductive and gynaecological morbidities *(369–378)*. Cases are often unreported or undocumented because people who are sexually assaulted often suffer feelings of shame, blame or psychological distress, and because the responses they get from formal institutions (police, judiciary, health), as well as from community members, are frequently unsympathetic, discriminatory and traumatizing. Very few cases of rape, for example, are actually reported to the police, making it almost impossible to estimate the actual extent of rape worldwide *(350)*, but it occurs in all countries of the world, both within and outside marriage and intimate partnerships. It is also widespread in times of conflict *(349)*.

The legal understanding of sexual assault and rape has been historically narrow in scope. Rape, for example, has traditionally been understood as "unlawful" sexual intercourse by a man with a woman who is not his wife, through force and against her will *(379)*, and involving vaginal penetration by a penis. Under such a definition, women who have been raped by their husbands, women who have been raped anally, men and transgender individuals cannot legitimately claim to have been raped. In 2010, international criminal law elaborated the elements of the crime of rape, radically changing this traditional understanding, and these elements have been affirmed by a number of national laws. The consideration of these elements requires, for example, a broader definition of what constitutes rape, which should cover coercive "invasion" or "conduct resulting in penetration, however slight, of any part of the body of the victim ... with a sexual organ, or of the anal or genital opening of the victim with any object or any other part of the body" *(380)*. The definition of rape should also be broad enough to be gender-neutral, meaning that it can apply to any person of whatever sex or gender *(380)*.

In addition, international and regional human rights laws now recognizes that rape can take place within marriage and is a crime in all circumstances (381). At the regional level, the language of the Protocol to the African Charter on Human and Peoples' Rights on the Rights of Women in Africa clearly indicates that immunity cannot be granted to husbands, as states are enjoined to adopt laws that prohibit "all forms of violence against women, including unwanted or forced sex whether the violence takes place in private or in public" *(37)*. In a similar vein, the European Court of Human Rights has ruled unacceptable the idea of a husband being immune to prosecution for raping his wife, in line with what the Court termed a civilized concept of marriage but also with the fundamental right of respect for human dignity *(382)*.

Many national laws have been amended over the past decade in line with these human rights standards. For example, laws have been changed to recognize that marital rape is a crime *(368)*; that rape can be committed by a person of any gender against another person of any gender; that any act of penetration can be considered as rape; and that evidence of physical force is not required as proof of rape (e.g. South Africa, Thailand; *383, 384*).

According to international human rights standards, the definition of rape should no longer require corroboration of a victim's testimony by third parties *(385)*. In this way, it can no longer be implied that women's testimony cannot be relied upon. Several national courts and legislatures have removed the requirement for corroboration of a third party to "prove" that rape has taken place. The South African Supreme Court, for example, specifically stated that such a requirement was "based on an irrational and out-dated perception and unjust stereotyping

against women as unreliable victims" *(386)*, and the Kenyan Court of Appeal found that such requirement constitutes discrimination against women and is contrary to the concept of equality *(387)*.

People held in detention, such as prisoners, can be particularly at risk of sexual violence, and those who are sex workers, homosexuals or transgender, as well as sex offenders, may be at increased risk of sexual violence from other inmates and sometimes also directly from prison guards *(388–390)*. Prison authorities' discriminatory attitudes towards these populations can create a climate in which such violations can easily proliferate *(121, 391)*.

Rape in custodial situations has been regarded as a form of torture and cruel, inhuman and degrading treatment *(390)*, and rape of a detainee by an official of the state is considered to be an especially grave and abhorrent form of ill treatment, given the ease with which the offender can exploit the vulnerability of his victim *(365)*. Based on human rights standards, states are called upon to design and implement appropriate measures to prevent all sexual violence in all detention centres, ensure that all allegations of violence in detention centres are investigated promptly and independently, that perpetrators are prosecuted and appropriately sentenced, and that victims can seek redress including appropriate compensation *(389, 390)*.

Some countries have established specific legal protections against prison rape. In the USA, for example, following data collection that confirmed that sexual abuse was a significant problem in prisons, jails and immigrant detention centres, and even more likely in juvenile facilities, a number of standards have been put in place *(392)*, including prohibition of the hiring or promotion of staff who have been engaged in coercive sex, and limits on body searches by opposite-sex staff *(388)*.

5.2.2 Sexual abuse of children

Sexual abuse of children (i.e. people under the age of 18) occurs in all regions of the world and is part of a broader phenomenon of child maltreatment *(393)*. It is a serious violation of a child's rights to health and protection. Evidence from different parts of the world indicates that up to 20% of women and

5–10% of men report having been sexually abused as children *(393, 394)*. Sexual abuse of children has not been well documented at a population level, but clinic-based studies have shown severe effects on health, including sexual health, such as injuries, STIs (including HIV), trauma, depression, anxiety and even death. In older female children, it may result in unwanted pregnancy and unsafe abortion with potential complications *(395)*. Sexually abused children are at increased risk for behavioural, physical and mental health problems including depression, smoking, obesity, high-risk sexual behaviours, harmful use of alcohol and drugs, and perpetrating or being a victim of violence *(368, 372, 393, 396–401)*.

Children are understood to be at risk of sexual harm in part because they lack the ability to claim their rights, and also in part because of the power imbalances between younger and older persons. International and regional human rights standards provide the framework for states' obligations to take all appropriate legislative, administrative, social and educational measures to protect children from all forms of physical or mental violence, injury or abuse, including sexual abuse *(34, 339, 402)* and to punish the perpetrators of such acts and protect the rights and interests of child victims *(403)*.

Regional standards also encourage children's participation, according to their evolving capacity, in the design and implementation of relevant state policies, stressing that assistance to victims shall take due account of the child's views, needs and concerns, and always take into account the best interests of the child. Importantly, the Convention on the Rights of the Child makes clear that it is not intended "to criminalize sexual activities of young adolescents who are discovering their sexuality and engaging in sexual experiences with each other in the framework of sexual development. Nor is it intended to cover sexual activities between persons of similar ages and maturity" *(402)*.

In the context of the rights of adolescents to health and development, international human rights bodies call on states to ensure that specific legal provisions are guaranteed under national law, including the possibility of accessing health services without parental consent. These provisions should closely reflect the recognition of the status of people under 18 years of age as rights holders, in accordance with their evolving capacity, age and maturity *(31, 40)*.

5.2.3 Forced marriage and sexual and sexuality-related violence

In a number of countries, children and adults – particularly women – may not be able to freely enter into marriage with their full consent for reasons linked to historical subordination, lack of economic independence, sociocultural tradition or family interest *(292)*. Practices related to forced marriage include child or early marriage, forced marriage in war, conflict and post-conflict situations, widow inheritance, and forced marriage with an abductor or rapist.

All such practices have a detrimental effect on the health and well-being of the people involved, and violate fundamental human rights. International human rights standards are unequivocal: "marriage shall be entered into only with the free and full consent of the intending spouses" *(32, 89, 326, 404, 405)*. Human rights bodies have frequently condemned both early and forced marriage as a violation of women's rights and have affirmed that a woman's right to choose when, if and whom she will marry must be protected and enforced by the law *(37, 110)*.

Child or early marriage. The practice of child or early marriage is widespread and occurs in all regions of the world. It prevents individuals from living their lives free from all forms of violence and it has adverse consequences on the enjoyment of human rights, such as the right to education, and the right to the highest attainable standard of health, including sexual and reproductive health *(406, 407)*.

Within marriage, young women and girls in particular are at risk of sexual abuse, rape, premature motherhood and domestic violence, with all associated physiological and psychological trauma *(348)*. Adolescent and child wives are less able than their adult counterparts to negotiate sex, or to make free and informed decisions affecting their sexual and reproductive health, including access to health services for contraception and the prevention and treatment of STIs *(408, 409)*.

Early marriage is very often linked to early childbearing as in many countries there is considerable pressure on girls to become pregnant soon after they are married *(410, 411)*. The health risks of early pregnancy for adolescent girls are considerable. Early childbirth is nearly always associated with lower socioeconomic status, reduced access to antenatal care, and poor nutritional status, all of which can lead to poor maternal and child health outcomes *(412–417)*. These include increased risks of: anaemia, premature labour, complications during delivery (including obstetric fistula), maternal death, low birth weight, and neonatal death *(412, 414, 418–420)*.

International and regional human rights standards and consensus documents call for the elimination of early and forced marriage *(37, 110, 406, 421)*. They call for the recognition of a minimum age of marriage, which should be 18 years for both men and women *(37, 110, 339)*, and for the official registration of all marriages to be compulsory *(339)*. They recognize the necessity of collective efforts of governments, lawmakers, judicial authorities, law enforcement officials, traditional and religious leaders, civil society, media, the private sector and other relevant stakeholders to address the root causes of this practice *(406)*.

In order to protect children and eliminate early marriage, most countries have put in place an enabling legal framework, setting the minimum age of marriage at 18 years in accordance with these human rights standards. Even in those countries, however, compliance is often poor for a variety of reasons, such as the lack of accurate registration of all births, which is necessary for establishing the age of those marrying, or the fact that many families remain financially and otherwise materially invested in early marriage practices *(419)*. National courts are increasingly responding to this practice, upholding the fundamental rights of women to consent to marriage *(422, 423)*. For example, a Sharia Court in Nigeria ruled that a marriage of a teenage girl conducted without her consent constituted a violation of the rights to liberty and dignity under the Nigerian Constitution and that it was against their understanding of Sharia Law *(423)*.

Forced marriage in conflict settings. Forced marriages arise in war, conflict and post-conflict settings where women, sometimes very young, are captured by fighters and forced to live as their "wives" (i.e. as sexual and/or domestic partners), essentially in slavery. Human rights bodies are calling for the elimination of such practices. In Sierra Leone, for example, forced marriage has been judged a crime against humanity, and is recognized as "resulting in severe suffering, or physical, mental or psychological injury to the victim" *(424)*.

Widow inheritance. Women's free and full consent to marriage is also infringed by the practice of widow inheritance in some places. Drawn from local customary law and religious practices, such marriages still occurs in some parts of Asia *(425)* and Africa *(426)*, although it is diminishing *(427)*. A surviving widow, whether a minor or an adult, is "inherited" by a male relative (often the brother) of the deceased spouse, along with other goods and property of the estate, such that she becomes his wife. Often this is the condition imposed on the widow for being able to remain in her house, or to receive support from her husband's kin *(427)*. Thus, she must enter a sexual relationship with a spouse not chosen by her, which is a form of coerced sex, with many potential negative sexual and reproductive health consequences *(428)*.

Under human rights laws, states have an obligation to end any practice whereby a widow is liable to be inherited by another person *(429)*, and states must ensure that "widows are not subjected to inhuman, humiliating or degrading treatment" and that a "widow shall have the right to remarry, and in that event, to marry the person of her choice" *(37)*.

Marriage with an abductor or rapist. Women may also be forced to marry against their will or without free and full consent in places where there are laws that allow mitigation (or complete annulment) of punishment for an abductor or rapist if he agrees to marry the woman he has abducted or raped. Such laws are discriminatory as well as being harmful to the well-being of the abducted or raped woman, as she is then pressured to take as her husband a person who has assaulted her. While a number of countries have such laws, there have been some positive reforms in line with international human rights protections, as, for example, in Ethiopia, which reformed its 1957 Penal Code in 2005 to remove the exculpation of an alleged rapist in light of a subsequent marriage to a victim *(430)*.

5.2.4. Violence based on real or perceived sexual behaviour or expression

Violence committed against persons because of their real or perceived sexual behaviour or expression has been recorded in all regions of the world *(121)*. Among these sexual behaviours or forms of sexual expression are: having same-sex sexual partner(s), having extramarital sex, engaging in sex work, perceived effeminate behaviour by men, sexual contact with those viewed as being social inferiors or members of enemy groups, behaviour deemed to dishonour the kin group, and sexual disobedience. These behaviours are perceived as being nonconformist, transgressing societal or moral codes or norms, and violence is used to punish people for such conduct. The violent punishment may be physical or psychological, and the effects include: injury, reduced ability to access treatment for these injuries, humiliation, disempowerment and increased disease burden *(121)*.

Violence based on sexual orientation or gender identity. There is increasing documentation of targeted violence against people who have (or are suspected to have) same-sex sexual relationships, and against transgender people. The extent of such violence is currently impossible to estimate as few states have systems in place for monitoring, recording and reporting these incidents. Even where systems exist, incidents may go unreported or are misreported because victims distrust the police, are afraid of reprisals or threats to privacy, or are stigmatized *(121)*.

Homophobic and transphobic violence can take many forms, including harassment and bullying in schools, so-called street violence and other spontaneous attacks in public settings *(121)*. Homophobic and transphobic violence can involve a high degree of cruelty and brutality, including beatings, murder, torture, rape and other types of sexual assault *(73, 121, 178, 201, 431, 432)*. Violent acts may be committed by family members and

friends, peers at school, health-care providers, co-workers, the police or others *(98, 121, 175, 201, 202, 207, 229, 433, 434)*.

Severe violence and torture occurring in health-care settings has been documented, including denial of medical treatment, use of verbal abuse and public humiliation, and a variety of forced procedures such as psychiatric evaluation and sterilization. Other types of violence perpetrated by health personnel and other state officials include forcible anal examination for the prosecution of suspected homosexual activities, invasive virginity examination, hormone therapy, and so-called sex normalizing surgery and reparative therapy. These procedures are rarely medically necessary, can cause serious injury, scarring, loss of sexual sensation, pain, incontinence and lifelong depression, and have also been criticized as being unscientific, potentially harmful and contributing to stigma *(178)*.

Lesbian, gay and transgender people may be subject to aggravated violence and abuse by inmates and prison guards when they are in detention or under state care *(121, 228, 229, 232, 435)*. Incidents have been reported in which individuals were subjected to victimization by police and prison guards, and authorities failed to take reasonable measures to prevent violence against detainees perceived as being lesbian, gay or transgender *(121)*.

Criminalization of same-sex sexual behaviour and non-gender-conforming behaviour, and discriminatory laws and regulations, can create and intensify stigma, discrimination and violence, all of which have direct effects on lesbian, gay, transgender, gender variant and intersex people's health far beyond immediate injury. Criminal laws, public decency regulations and policing surveillance systems have all been used to harass, arrest, torture, rape and abuse people perceived as belonging to these groups *(121, 435–437)*.

International and regional human rights bodies increasingly call for the respect and protection of lesbian, gay, transgender, gender variant and intersex people's human rights, including respect for their rights to life, liberty and security of person, to be free from torture or inhuman and degrading

treatment and discrimination, the rights to privacy, freedom of expression, association and peaceful assembly, and the right to the highest attainable standard of health (107, 121, 175, 183, 184, 242, 363, 434, 438). They have also recognized that stigma, discrimination, marginalization and violence related to sexual orientation and gender identity and expression are often exacerbated by other personal characteristics and factors, such as race, ethnicity, religion, socioeconomic status, being a migrant or residing in conflict settings, and so they have called for the elimination of multiple discrimination (107, 178, 210, 242 [paragraph 18]).

International and regional human rights bodies have clearly condemned violent crime perpetrated against persons because of their sexual orientation and/or gender identity and expression, including by law enforcement officials, as well as the failure of states to address such crime in their legislation (121, 439). They have urged states to ensure that these acts of violence and human rights violations are investigated and their perpetrators brought to justice (184, 440). Human rights bodies call on states to adopt legislation and public policies against discrimination and violence by reason of gender identity and expression (121, 434). They have also called for the implementation of special measures – including appropriate training of law enforcement and judicial officials – to protect persons in prison against bias-motivated crimes related to their sexual orientation or gender identity (390, 440).

A number of countries in all regions address discrimination and violence on the basis of sexual orientation and gender identity in their legislation (121, 175). Some have included provisions in their laws for addressing crimes committed on the basis of sexual orientation and gender identity, and included hate crimes and bias-motivated crimes related to sexual orientation and gender identity and expression in the hate crimes statute (e.g. Australia, USA; 441, 442). The anti-discrimination law in Serbia, for example, establishes the fundamental principle of equality of people of different sexes and genders, and includes sexual orientation and gender identity among the grounds for non-discrimination (443). It specifies that rights pertaining to gender or gender

change cannot be denied either publicly or privately, and it prohibits any physical violence, exploitation, expression of hatred, disparagement, blackmail and harassment pertaining to gender (443).

Honour crimes and honour killings. In some regions, people may be killed because they are seen by family or community members as having brought shame or dishonour on a family, often for transgressing gender norms or for sexual behaviour, including actual or assumed same-sex sexual activity (444–447). Documented crimes committed in the name of honour are most often perpetrated against women because of relations with a male partner who is viewed as an unacceptable match, or because of actual or assumed sex before marriage; one estimate suggests that at least 5000 women around the world are murdered by family members each year in these so-called honour killings (448). However, such crimes may also be committed against men and transgender people. Very often, these crimes remain unpunished and at times are even sanctioned by the law.

International human rights bodies have stated that these crimes violate the rights to life, to equality before the law, and to equal protection in the law, and have strongly recommend that states pass legislation "to remove the defence of honour in regard to the assault or murder of a female family member" (292). At the national level, some countries have changed their laws to reflect these human rights standards. In Turkey, for instance, where so-called honour killings were previously tolerated or even condoned by the state, a change in the Penal Code now takes the "honour" element of a killing as an aggravating instead of a mitigating factor in a criminal trial, signalling that such notions are a violation of human rights (449).

Eligibility for asylum. People who have fled their country for fear of hate crimes or honour killings may be eligible for asylum in states that have ratified the 1951 Refugee Convention. According to this Convention, states must not expel or return a refugee to a place where their life or freedom would be threatened on account of race, religion, nationality, political opinion or membership of a particular social group (450). Individuals who fear hate crimes or honour killings, including on account of their sexual orientation or gender identity, and where one cannot call on the state to provide protection from that harm, may be considered members of a "particular social group" *(451)*. The European Union, for example, has issued a legally binding directive providing protection for refugees on similar grounds *(452)* and some national-level laws and policies also reflect such protection (e.g. the USA; *453*).

United Nations guidance issued to Member States in relation to implementing the Refugee Convention and its 1967 Protocol also provides for the possibility of claims by women, men and transgender people based on fear of persecution on grounds related to sexual and sexuality-related violence *(115, 451)*. The 2008 guideline issued by the United Nations High Commissioner for Refugees (UNHCR) recommends that Member States should consider revising their laws to support refugee status, including asylum, for people who are persecuted for their sexual conduct, whatever its nature and whether it is real or perceived. Persecution includes prosecution under national laws, particularly when punishments include threats to life and bodily integrity or contribute to discrimination, and applies to people who may be persecuted for same-sex sexual conduct *(451)*.

5.2.5 Violence against people engaged in sex work

Around the world, people engaged in sex work are subjected to high levels of harassment and violence *(454)*. Such violence is often perpetrated by law enforcement authorities as well as by clients (or people posing as clients), pimps, managers of sex work establishments, and intimate partners *(455–458)*. Police violence and harassment, including coercion to provide sex to police in exchange for release from detainment or to avoid fines *(290, 457, 459)*, is reported by people engaged in sex work in many regions *(289, 460–463)*. Because of this, people engaged in sex work report that they would be unlikely to go to the police for help if they were raped or suffered other forms of violence *(461, 464)*. Thus they have little recourse to police protection and little hope that violence and other crimes against them will be investigated *(284, 462, 465–468)*.

This environment of violence committed with impunity leads to myriad vulnerabilities. First, even if condoms are available, people engaged in sex work may be unable to use them – either because the sexual encounter is coerced (rape) or because the law or police practice creates a situation in which it is not possible to negotiate condom use. In some places, the mere fact of carrying condoms may be used as evidence to support criminal charges relating to sex work *(469, 470)*. Secondly, aggressive policing may drive sex workers away from familiar areas with informal support networks to places where they are more isolated, less able to negotiate with clients, more vulnerable to violence *(277, 455, 457, 459, 463, 471, 472)* and less able to access health services *(285, 473, 474)*. Wherever sex work is effectively criminalized, clients' knowledge that they cannot be reported to the police by a sex worker makes the sex workers additionally vulnerable to violence *(461, 464)*.

Some studies show that where the brothel industry is legally regulated – such that safety and health conditions for sex workers and their clients are guaranteed – violence against people engaged in sex work is dramatically less in brothels than in non-brothel venues *(475, 476)* and corruption or organized crime is minimized *(477)*. Such safety conditions can include requirements for the installation of easily accessible alarm buttons in all rooms used for sex work *(478)* and assurances that sex workers can refuse to provide sexual services if they believe the situation is potentially unsafe *(295)*.

Human rights standards call for non-discrimination and protection from violence of people engaged in sex work *(73)*. States must ensure, at a minimum, that women in sex work are free from violence or discrimination, whether by state agents or private persons, and that they have access to equal protection of the law. The health needs and rights of women engaged in sex work require special attention, particularly where their illegal status renders them vulnerable to violence *(28, 73, 292)*. According to international human rights law and standards, forcible or fraudulent movement into sex work is a violation of human rights and is prohibited *(15, 293)*.

5.2.6 Trafficking for forced prostitution

Trafficking for forced prostitution,[11] like other types of forced labour, occurs in all regions of the world. It has been recognized as a major human rights violation and is known to have an extensive impact on both the sexual health and general health of those who are trafficked. Accurate statistics on the magnitude of human trafficking are elusive, due as much to different definitions still in use in some countries as to its illegal nature, but trafficking of adults and children for forced prostitution or other forms of forced labour has been documented in over 137 countries in the world (479).

Under international law, the crime of trafficking is held to be "the recruitment, transportation, transfer, harbouring or receipt of persons, by means of the threat or use of force or other forms of coercion, of abduction, of fraud, of deception, of the abuse of power or of a position of vulnerability or of the giving or receiving of payments or benefits to achieve the consent of a person having control over another person, for the purpose of exploitation. Exploitation shall include, at a minimum, the exploitation of the prostitution of others or other forms of sexual exploitation, forced labour or services, slavery or practices similar to slavery, servitude or the removal of organs" (15). United Nations standards leave it up to states to decide whether or not to criminalize the non-coercive buying and selling of sex. However, they clearly define the movement of people under 18 into prostitution as a trafficking crime (15).

In addition to the physical and mental trauma of being trafficked, those who are trafficked for forced prostitution are exposed to coerced and forced sex, and are unable to refuse sex or to use or negotiate the use of condoms, thus putting them at risk of acquiring STIs including HIV (480–484), and gynaecological problems, such as vaginal discharge, pelvic pain and infection, as well as headaches, back pains, fatigue, depression and post-traumatic stress

disorder (480, 482–484). Persons who are trafficked for other reasons, such as for domestic work, may also be abused sexually as this is a common tactic used by traffickers to intimidate trafficked persons in any labour sector (479). Because of their sequestered and often illegal situation, trafficked persons often have no opportunity to move freely or get information and they may be denied access to health and social services, including sexual health services (480, 484). The reluctance or inability of the trafficked individuals to report or denounce any form of abuse to authorities, for fear of the consequences related to their illegal or irregular immigration status, further increases their vulnerability (480). As with other forms of sexual violence, more data are available on women and girls than on men, boys and transgender people.

Nearly all states criminalize some forms of trafficking and most forms of forced labour. Laws such as the law in Thailand, for example, require the provision of specific assistance for trafficked people including the provision of food, shelter, medical treatment, physical and mental rehabilitation, education, training and legal aid (485).

International and regional human rights bodies and other institutions of the United Nations have called on states to take all appropriate measures to suppress all forms of trafficking, including putting in place laws to penalize those who traffic people (15), and special attention has been paid to women (34, 37, 326, 486). International human rights law also makes it clear that any measures adopted to prevent trafficking should not restrict fundamental rights of those trafficked, such as the right to non-discrimination (15). To protect both the sexual health and human rights of those who have been trafficked into forced prostitution or other forced labour, states must also provide legal and other protections such as medical and psychological health services (including sexual health information, care and counselling) for those trafficked (15, 28, 487, 488). Human rights bodies also call for remedies for trafficked people, including their right to reparations. This should include access to information and legal assistance, and regularization of residence status (489).

---

11 Trafficking people into forced prostitution is not the same as sex work involving consenting adults. Sex work refers to a contractual arrangement where sexual services are negotiated between consenting adults with the terms of engagement agreed upon between the seller and the buyer (17).

Many children in the world are coerced or trafficked into prostitution *(490)*, which is not only a cause of serious ill health but is also a gross violation of children's rights. International and regional human rights standards stress that states must protect the child from all forms of sexual exploitation and sexual abuse, the exploitative use of children in prostitution or other unlawful sexual practices, and they urge states to take priority action in this regard *(34, 37, 303, 403)*.

5.2.7 Female genital mutilation

Female genital mutilation (FGM), a procedure involving partial or total removal of the external female genitalia or other injury to the female genital organs for non-medical reasons, has been classified as a type of violence against girls *(292)*. An estimated 100–140 million girls and women worldwide are estimated to have undergone such procedures and 3 million girls are estimated to be at risk of undergoing FGM every year *(94)*. FGM has been reported in all parts of the world, but its practice is most prevalent in the western, eastern and north-eastern regions of Africa, some countries in Asia and the Middle East, and among certain immigrant communities in North America and Europe *(94)*.

FGM has no known health benefits. On the contrary, it is known to be harmful to girls and women in many ways, including direct negative effects on sexuality and sexual health *(94)*. The removal of or damage to healthy, normal genital tissue interferes with the natural functioning of the body and causes several immediate and long-term health consequences. Almost all those who have undergone FGM experience pain and bleeding as a consequence of the procedure. The intervention itself can be traumatic as girls are often physically held down during the procedure *(491, 492)*. Even if performed in a hospital, the procedure can result in severe pain, shock, excessive bleeding, difficulty in passing urine, infections, psychological trauma and death *(94)*. Long-term consequences can include chronic pain, infections, decreased sexual enjoyment, and psychological consequences such as post-traumatic stress disorder *(94)*. Women who have undergone FGM are more likely to experience pain during sexual intercourse, experience significantly less sexual satisfaction and are twice as likely to report lack of

sexual desire, compared to women who have not undergone the procedure *(493)*.

FGM is used as a way of controlling female sexuality *(94)*. Some of the specific justifications offered for FGM are linked to girls' marriageability and are consistent with the characteristics considered necessary for a woman to become a proper wife. It is often believed that the practice ensures and preserves a girl's or woman's virginity *(492, 494–496)*. In some communities, it is thought to restrain sexual desire, thereby ensuring marital fidelity and preventing sexual behaviour that is considered deviant and immoral *(495, 497–499)*. FGM is also considered to make girls clean and beautiful. Removal of genital parts is thought to eliminate parts viewed as masculine, such as the clitoris *(496, 498, 500)* or, in the case of infibulation, to achieve smoothness, which is considered to be beautiful *(495, 496)*. A belief sometimes expressed by women is that FGM enhances men's sexual pleasure *(501)*. Any form of FGM reflects deep-rooted inequality between the sexes, and constitutes an extreme form of discrimination against women and girls.

FGM has been recognized as a form of violence and a harmful practice that violates well-established human rights principles, norms and standards, including the principles of equality and non-discrimination on the basis of sex, the right to life (when the procedure results in death), and the right to freedom from torture or cruel, inhuman or degrading treatment or punishment *(94)*. International and regional human rights standards characterize FGM as a form of gender-based violence and call upon states to take appropriate and effective measures to eliminate all forms of FGM *(37, 339, 502)* including the adoption of legislation and ensuring that perpetrators are brought before the courts *(503)*. Measures should also include the creation of public awareness in all sectors of society, including through education and outreach programmes, and the provision of support to victims of FGM and other harmful practices, including counselling, legal, vocational and health services *(37)*. The medicalization of FGM – that is, its practice by any health-care provider – should also be prohibited *(37, 504)*.

An increasing number of African countries have specific legislation to address FGM, along with policies and programmes involving community education and encouraging a process of positive social change (94). However, legal measures include punishments of varying severity and few convictions have occurred, and not all laws impose duties on the state to educate and raise awareness about the harmful effects of the practice (10).

Where FGM is a problem among immigrant communities, such as in Europe, North America and the Western Pacific, there is mostly strong condemnation by states and zero tolerance of FGM within the host country (8, 9, 13). As in Africa, the majority of anti-FGM efforts in Europe are to be found in criminal law with harsh prison sentences, which may have the effect of pushing the practice underground and stigmatizing girls and women further (505). Some preventive work is being undertaken, through child protection laws for instance (13), and in several countries, especially in Europe and North America, asylum may be granted to girls or women who would otherwise be forced to undergo FGM (13, 506, 507).

5.2.8 Coercive practices within health services that affect sexual health and sexuality

Coercive practices within health services related to sexual health have been documented in many parts of the world. These include the use of coercion for providing contraceptive methods such as implants and sterilization, forced abortion (508), and procedures such as virginity testing or forced HIV testing. The cases of coerced and forced sterilization and virginity testing are highlighted in this report to demonstrate the health dimensions and the extensive human rights standards that have been elaborated to address the problem.

Coerced and forced sterilization. Sterilization is one of the most widely used forms of contraception in the world. When performed according to appropriate clinical standards with informed consent, sterilization methods such as vasectomy and tubal ligation are safe and effective methods of permanently ending fertility. Like any other

contraceptive method, sterilization should only be provided with the full, free and informed consent of the individual. However, in some countries, persons belonging to certain population groups, including persons with disabilities, persons living with HIV, persons from ethnic minorities, transgender and intersex persons, continue to be sterilized without their free and informed consent. Other individuals may also be at risk of coercive sterilization, such as persons with a substance dependence and those engaged in sex work. Women and girls continue to be disproportionately impacted (91). Coercive sterilization was used as an instrument of population control, particularly during the period from the 1960s to the 1990s. Despite international agreements, in which states agreed to support the principle of voluntary choice in family planning, there are still some settings in which people from socially marginalized groups are subjected to involuntary sterilization as part of government strategies to reduce population growth (91).

International human rights and ethical bodies have explicitly condemned coercive population policies and programmes. They note that decisions about sterilization should not be subject to arbitrary requirements imposed by a governmental body (78, 509, 510) and that states' obligations to protect persons from such treatment extends into the private sphere, including where such practices are committed by private individuals (363). Coerced and/or forced sterilization of women has also been characterized as a form of discrimination and violence against women (28, 292, 509, 511, 512) and a violation of their rights to health, information and privacy, as well as their rights to decide on the number and spacing of children, to found a family, and to be free from torture or inhuman and degrading treatment (40, 169, 292, 389, 513–518). Human rights bodies have also recognized that coerced sterilization can constitute torture and other cruel, inhuman or degrading treatment or punishment, and that coerced sterilization committed as part of a widespread or systematic attack on any civilian population constitutes a crime against humanity (14, 519).

Female virginity testing. In some parts of the world, female virginity is considered a precondition for marriage, and some marriage traditions include practices to confirm that the bride is a virgin. This is often done through the tradition of showing to the bride and groom's families the blood-stained sheets after the wedding night *(520)*. Virginity testing covers a variety of practices to test whether a girl or woman has had sexual intercourse, based on the belief that female virginity can be reliably and unambiguously verified. These tests can be highly intrusive, and not only are they degrading, humiliating and painful for the woman involved but also detrimental to her reproductive and sexual health. For example, the emphasis on virginity may divert attention from the need for safer sex practices and information about risks to sexual health; anal sex may replace vaginal sex before marriage, because it seems "safe" from the perspective of appearing to preserve virginity and avoiding pregnancy, but it can be unsafe in terms of sexual transmission of infections, including HIV. Furthermore, female virginity testing is a violation of the right to non-discrimination, the right to physical and psychological integrity, the right to respect for one's private life, and the right not to be subjected to cruel, inhuman and degrading treatment *(56, 521, 522)*. Some national courts have upheld these human rights standards. In Nepal, for example, the Supreme Court recognized women's right to have control over their own bodies when it nullified the Virginity Test Order of Kathmandu District Court in 1998 *(523)*.

5.3 Conclusion

Sexual violence and sexuality-related violence occur in all parts of the world. Some people may be especially vulnerable to such violence, including women, children, people in custodial situations, people with disabilities, and/or people whose real or perceived sexual orientation or gender identity is deemed unacceptable. Violence in any form is detrimental to mental and physical health and other aspects of well-being.

Sexual and sexuality-related violence includes, but is not limited to, sexual assault and rape, forced and early marriage, trafficking into forced prostitution, harmful traditional practices such as FGM, and honour killings. Such violence takes place in intimate personal environments, such as marriage and domestic settings, and is also used as a weapon of war in conflict settings. Often it is committed by people in positions of authority and responsibility for the safety and well-being of others, for example in detention facilities. In health-care settings, violence that has an impact on sexual health includes forced sterilization and forced virginity testing. Health-care providers may inflict violence on their patients because of their real or perceived sexual orientation or gender identity.

Different forms of sexual and sexuality-related violence are violations of human rights. In accordance with human rights standards, states must adopt legislative, administrative, social, economic and other measures necessary to prevent, investigate and punish acts of violence including all forms of sexual violence, whether perpetrated by the state or by private persons, and they must provide support and assistance to the victims of violence, including access to health services. States should also provide effective remedies, compensation and mechanisms for seeking redress. This obligation applies with respect to all persons, regardless of their sex, gender, age, sexual orientation, gender identity, marital or other status, and irrespective of who it was that committed violence against them, in whatever context. Laws can play an important role in fostering the recognition of all forms of violence as a human rights violation and a crime. They can be crucial in setting guarantees and frameworks for government actions to prevent, eliminate and deal with the consequences of violence, and a number of countries in different regions have developed laws in line with these human rights standards.

5.4 Legal and policy implications

On the basis of the human rights standards described in this chapter, and in order to safeguard sexual health and well-being, the following questions should be examined by those who are responsible for setting enabling legal and policy frameworks.

1. Has the state adopted legislative and all other measures necessary to prevent, investigate and punish acts of violence, including all forms of sexual violence, whether perpetrated by the state or by private persons? Are there provisions for the state to provide effective remedies, compensation and mechanisms for seeking redress, for all persons?

2. Do national laws provide a broad definition of sexual assault and rape that includes gender-neutral language (committed by a person of any gender against a person of any gender), and which recognizes that sexual assault and rape can take place in martial relationships and in custodial situations, and that third-party testimony is not required as proof of the crime?

3. Do national laws provide specific protection for children against sexual abuse?

4. Is violence, whether specifically sexual or non-sexual, committed against people who are perceived to transgress sexual and/or gender norms recognized as a violation of their human rights? Has the state put in place protections for all people on the basis of non-discrimination?

5. Do laws contain provisions that guarantee the protection of human rights for people engaged in sex work?

6. Has the state taken all legal measures to penalize those who traffic people including into forced prostitution, as well as to provide protective measures and health services to victims of trafficking?

7. Has the state taken appropriate and effective measures to eliminate FGM, through both legislation as well as education and public awareness campaigns? Does it provide support to the victims of FGM, including counselling, legal, vocational and health services, as well as other measures to protect girls and women who are at risk, including prohibiting the medicalization of the practice?

8. Does the state recognize that forced sterilization or other coerced or forced procedures affecting sexual and reproductive health are a violation of human rights? Has it put in place measures to protect people against such forced interventions?

9. Do laws and/or policies ensure participation of various stakeholders and affected populations with regard to the elaboration of laws, policies, programmes and services related to health services/ health information and education/violence?

References

1. Developing sexual health programmes: a framework for action. Geneva: World Health Organization; 2010.

2. Education and treatment in human sexuality: the training of health professionals. Technical Report Series, No. 572. Geneva: World Health Organization; 1975.

3. Programme of Action of the International Conference on Population and Development (ICPD). New York (NY): United Nations; 1994.

4. Defining sexual health: report of a technical consultation on sexual health, 28–31 January 2002. Geneva: World Health Organization; 2006.

5. Reproductive health strategy to accelerate progress towards the attainment of international development goals and targets. Geneva: World Health Organization; 2004.

6. Baghat H, Boutros M. Using human rights for sexuality and sexual health: Eastern Mediterranean region. Working paper commissioned by the World Health Organization. International Council on Human Rights Policy; 2010.

7. Bhardwaj K, Divan V. Sexual health and human rights: a legal and jurisprudential review of select countries in the SEARO region – Bangladesh, India, Indonesia, Nepal, Sri Lanka and Thailand. Working paper commissioned by the World Health Organization. International Council on Human Rights Policy; 2011 (http://www.ichrp.org/files/papers/182/140_searo_divan_bhardwaj_2011.pdf, accessed 5 February 2015).

8. Cusack S. Advancing sexual health and human rights in the Western Pacific. Working paper commissioned by the World Health Organization. International Council on Human Rights Policy; 2010 (http://www.ichrp.org/files/papers/179/140_Simone_Cusack_Western_Pacific_2010.pdf, accessed 5 February 2015).

9. Miller AM, Roseman MJ, Friedman C. Sexual health and human rights: United States and Canada. Working paper commissioned by the World Health Organization. International Council on Human Rights Policy; 2010 (http://www.ichrp.org/files/papers/178/140_Miller_Roseman_Friedman_uscan_2010.pdf, accessed 30 June 2013).

10. Ngwena C. Sexual health and human rights in the African region. Working paper commissioned by the World Health Organization. International Council on Human Rights Policy; 2011 (http://www.ichrp.org/files/papers/185/140_Ngwena_Africa_2011.pdf, accessed 5 January 2015).

11. Restrepo-Saldarriaga E. Advancing sexual health through human rights in Latin America and the Caribbean. Working paper commissioned by the World Health Organization. International Council on Human Rights Policy; 2010 (http://www.ichrp.org/files/papers/183/140_Restrepo_LAC_2011.pdf, accessed 21 January 2015).

12. Roseman M, Miller A. International legal norms/standards related to sexual health. Working paper commissioned by the World Health Organization. 2011 (unpublished).

13. Westeson J. Sexual health and human rights: European region. Working paper commissioned by the World Health Organization. International Council on Human Rights Policy; 2010 (http://www.ichrp.org/files/papers/177/140_Johanna_Westeson_Europe_2010.pdf, accessed 5 February 2015).

14. Rome Statute of the International Criminal Court. New York (NY): United Nations; 1998.

15. Protocol to prevent, suppress and punish trafficking in persons, especially women and children, supplementing the United Nations Convention against Transnational Organized Crime. New York (NY): United Nations; 2000.

16. Handbook and guidelines on procedures and criteria for determining refugee status under the 1951 Convention and the 1967 Protocol relating to the status of refugees. Geneva: United Nations High Commissioner for Refugees; 2011.

17. Global Commission on HIV and the Law. HIV and the law: risks, rights and health. New York (NY): United Nations Development Programme; 2012.

18. Global report. UNAIDS report on the global AIDS epidemic 2013. Geneva: Joint United Nations Programme on HIV/AIDS (UNAIDS); 2013.

19. Prevalence and incidence of selected sexually transmitted infections: Chlamydia trachomatis, *Neisseria gonorrhoeae*, syphilis and *Trichomonas vaginalis*. Geneva: World Health Organization; 2011.

20. Guttmacher Institute. Facts on investing in family planning and maternal and newborn health. New York (NY): Guttmacher Institute; 2010.

21. Prevention and treatment of HIV and other sexually transmitted infections among men who have sex with men and transgender people. Recommendation for a public health approach. Geneva: World Health Organization; 2011.

22. Feyisetan B, Caseterline C. Fertility preferences and contraceptive change in developing countries. New York (NY): Population Council; 2004.

23. Reducing risks by offering contraceptive services. New York (NY): United Nations Population Fund; 2011 (http://www.unfpa.org/public/cache/offonce/home/mothers/pid/4382, accessed 1 May 2014).

24. Harper CC, Cheong M, Rossa CH, Darney PD, Raine TR. The effect of increased access to emergency contraception among young adolescents. Obstet Gynecol. 2005;106(3):483–91.

25. Gold MA, Wolford JE, Smith KA, Parker AM. The effects of advance provision of emergency contraception on adolescent women's sexual and contraceptive behaviors. J Pediatr Adolesc Gynecol. 2004;17(2):87–96.

26. Krishnamurti T, Eggers SL, Fischhoff B. The impact of over-the-counter availability of « Plan B » on teens' contraceptive decision making. Soc Sci Med. 2008;67(4):618–27.

27. Cancer information sheet: sex, erectile dysfunction and prostate cancer. Dublin: Irish Cancer Society; 2011.

28. General Recommendation No. 24: Article 12: Women and health. New York (NY): United Nations Committee on the Elimination of Discrimination against Women; 1999 (A/54/38/Rev.1, Chapter I).

29. General Comment No. 14: The right to the highest attainable standard of health (Article 12 of the Covenant). New York (NY): United Nations Committee on Economic, Social and Cultural Rights; 2000 (E/C.12/2000/4).

30. General Comment No. 16: The equal right of men and women to the enjoyment of all economic, social and cultural rights (art. 3 of the International Covenant on Economic, Social and Cultural Rights). New York (NY): United Nations Committee on Economic, Social and Cultural Rights; 2005 (E/C.12/2005/4).

31. General Comment No. 4: Adolescent health and development in the context of the Convention on the Rights of the Child. New York (NY): United Nations Committee on the Rights of the Child; 2003 (CRC/GC/2003/4).

32. International Covenant on Economic, Social and Cultural Rights. New York (NY): United Nations; 1966.

33. Resolution 34/180: Convention on the Elimination of All Forms of Discrimination against Women. Thirty-fourth session of the General Assembly, 18 December 1979. New York (NY): United Nations; 1979.

34. Convention on the Rights of the Child. General Assembly resolution 44/25 of 20 November 1989. New York (NY): United Nations; 1989 (Entry into force 2 September 1990).

35. Political Declaration on HIV/AIDS. United Nations General Assembly resolution 60/262 of 15 June 2006. New York (NY): United Nations; 2006.

36. Convention on the Rights of Persons with Disabilities. New York (NY): United Nations; 2007.

37. African Commission on Human and People's Rights. Protocol to the African Charter on Human and Peoples' Rights on the Rights of Women in Africa. Maputo: African Union; 2003 (http://www.achpr.org/files/instruments/women-protocol/achpr_instr_proto_women_eng.pdf, accessed 5 February 2015).

38. Constitution of the Republic of South Africa. No. 108 of 1996. Republic of South Africa; 1996.

39. Constituição da República Portuguesa [Constitution of the Portuguese Republic]. República Portuguesa; 2005 (in Portuguese).

40. General Comment No. 15: The rights of the child to the highest attainable standard of health. Geneva: United Nations Committee on the Rights of the Child; 2013 (CRC/C/GC/15).

41. General Comment No. 31: The nature of the general legal obligation imposed on States Parties to the Covenant. Geneva: United Nations Human Rights Committee; 2004 (CCPR/C/21/Rev.1/Add.13).

42. Views on Communication No. 17/2008: Alyne da Silva Pimentel Teixeira v. Brazil. Geneva: United Nations Committee on the Elimination of Discrimination against Women; 2011 (CEDAW/C/49/D/17/2008).

43. Medicines: essential medicines. Fact sheet No. 325. Geneva: World Health Organization; 2010.

44. Hogerzeil HV, Samson M, Casanovas JV, Rahmani-Ocora L. Is access to essential medicines as part of the fulfilment of the right to health enforceable through the courts? Lancet. 2006;368:305–11.

45. The selection and use of essential medicines. Technical Report Series, 920:54. Geneva: World Health Organization; 2003.

46. WHO Model List of Essential Medicines. 17th list. Geneva: World Health Organization; 2011.

47. Sentencia del 5 de junio de 2008. Exp. 11001-03-24-000-2002-00251-01, Boletín No. 25 – Junio 16/08. República de Colombia Consejo de Estado [Council of State of the Republic of Colombia]; 2008 (in Spanish).

48. Controversia Constitucional 54/2009, decided on 27 May 2010 (Section IV). Estados Unidos Mexicanos Suprema Corte de Justicia (Supreme Court of the United Mexican States); 2010 (in Spanish).

49. Sentencia 7435-2006-PC/TC, decided on 13 November 2006. Rebública del Perú Tribunal Constitucional [Constitutional Tribunal of the Republic of Peru]; 2006 (in Spanish).

50. Smeaton v. Secretary of State for Health. EWHC 610 (Admin), decided on 18 April 2002. England and Wales High Court of Justice; 2002.

51. Canada Health Act (R.S.C., 1985, c. C-6). Canada; 1985.

52. European standards on subsidizing contraceptives. Fact sheet. Center for Reproductive Rights; 2009.

53. Chavkin W, Leitman L, Polin K, for Global Doctors for Choice. Conscientious objection and refusal to provide reproductive healthcare: a white paper examining prevalence, health consequences, and policy responses. Int J Gynecol Obstet. 2013;123(Suppl 3):S41–S56.

54. Zampas C, Andion-Ibaniez X. Conscientious objection to sexual and reproductive health services: international human rights standards and European law and practice. Eur J Health Law. 2012;19(3):231–56.

55. Johnson BR Jr, Kismödi E, Dragoman MV, Temmerman M. Conscientious objection to provision of legal abortion care. Int J Gynecol Obstet. 2013;123(Suppl 3):S60–S62.

56. Yazgül Yilmaz v. Turkey. Application No. 36369/06, decided on 1 February 2011. Strasbourg: European Court of Human Rights; 2011.

57. P. and S. v. Poland. Application No. 57375/08, decided on 30 October 2012. Strasbourg: European Court of Human Rights; 2012.

58. FIGO Committee for the Ethical Aspects of Human Reproduction and Women's Health. Ethical guidelines on conscientious objection. Int J Gynecol Obstet. 2006;92(3):333–4.

59. Safe abortion: technical and policy guidance for health systems, revised edition. Geneva: World Health Organization; 2012.

60. Ensuring human rights in the provision of contraceptive information and services. Geneva: World Health Organization; 2014.

61. Concluding observations: Poland. New York (NY): United Nations Committee on the Elimination of Discrimination against Women; 2007 (CEDAW/C/POL/CO/6).

62. Concluding comments: Slovakia. New York (NY): United Nations Committee on the Elimination of Discrimination against Women; 2008 (CEDAW/C/SVK/CO).

63. Concluding observations: Portugal. New York (NY): United Nations Committee on the Elimination of Discrimination against Women; 2008 (CEDAW/C/PRT/CO/7).

64. Pichon and Sajous v. France. Application No. 49853/99, Admissibility decision, decided on 2 October 2001. Strasbourg: European Court of Human Rights; 2001.

65. Sexual and reproductive health core competencies in primary health care. Geneva: World Health Organization; 2011.

66. Task shifting to improve access to contraceptive methods. Geneva: World Health Organization; 2013.

67. Increasing women's use of the IUD for family planning. Program Brief No. 9. New York (NY): Population Council; 2008.

68. Farr G, Rivera R, Amatya R. Non-physician insertion of IUDs: clinical outcomes among TCu380A insertions in three developing-country clinics. Adv Contracept 1998;14(1):45–57.

69. Lassner KJ, Chen CHC, Kropsch LA, Oberle MW, Lopes IM, Morris L. Comparative study of safety and efficacy of IUD insertions by physicians and nursing personnel in Brazil. Bull Pan Am Health Organ. 1995;29(3):206–15.

70. Wright NH, Sujpluem C, Rosenfield AG, Varakamin S. Nurse-midwife insertion of copper T in Thailand: performance, acceptance, and programmatic effects. Stud Fam Plann. 1977;8(9):237–43.

71. Wright KL. IUD insertion by nurse-midwives increases use. Network. 2003;23(1):13.

72. Law No. 92 of 1996: Choice on Termination of Pregnancy Act. 1996. Republic of South Africa; 1996.

73. Report of the Special Rapporteur on the right of everyone to the enjoyment of the highest attainable standard of physical and mental health, Anand Grover. New York (NY): United Nations; 2010.

74. Report of the Special Rapporteur on the right of everyone to the enjoyment of the highest attainable standard of physical and mental health. New York (NY): United Nations General Assembly; 2011.

75. Joyce TJ, Henshaw SK, Dennis A, Finer LB, Blanchard K. The impact of state mandatory counselling and waiting period laws on abortion: a literature review. New York (NY): Guttmacher Institute; 2009.

76. Payne D. More British abortions for Irish women. BMJ. 1999;318(7176):77.

77. Concluding observations of the Committee on the Rights of the Child: Chile. Third periodic report. New York (NY): United Nations; 2007 (CRC/C/CHL/CO/3).

78. General Comment No. 28: The equality of rights between men and women. Geneva: United Nations Human Rights Committee; 2000 (CCPR/C/21/Rev.1/Add.10).

79. Report of the Committee on the Elimination of Discrimination against Women. Twenty-second session and twenty-third session. New York (NY): United Nations; 2000 (A/55/38 (Supp) Chapter IV. Consideration of reports submitted by States Parties under article 18 of the Convention. Section B.2. Initial and second periodic reports of Jordan).

80. Arends-Kuenning M, Kessy FL. The impact of demand factors, quality of care and access to facilities on contraceptive use in Tanzania. J Biosoc Sci. 2007; 39(1):1–26.

81. Koenig MA. The impact of quality of care on contraceptive use: evidence from longitudinal data from rural Bangladesh. Baltimore (MD): Johns Hopkins University; 2003.

82. RamaRao S, Lacuesta M, Costello M, Pangolibay B, Jones H. The link between quality of care and contraceptive use. Int Perspect Sex Reprod Health. 2003;29(2):76–83.

83. Sanogo D, RamaRao S, Jones H, N'diaye P, M'bow B, Diop CB. Improving quality of care and use of contraceptives in Senegal. Afr J Reprod Health. 2003;7(2):57–73.

84. General Comment No. 3: HIV/AIDS and the rights of the child. New York (NY): United Nations Committee on the Rights of the Child; 2003 (CRC/GC/2003/03).

85. Cook RJ, Dickens BM, Fathalla M. Reproductive health and human rights: integrating medicine, ethics, and law. Oxford: Clarendon Press; 2003.

86. Klein J, Wilson K, McNulty M. Access to medical care for adolescents: results from the 1997 Commonwealth Fund Survey of the Health of Adolescent Girls. J Adolesc Health. 1999;25:120–30.

87. Lehrer JA, Pantell JA, Tebb K, Shafer MA. Forgone health care among US adolescents: associations between risk characteristics and confidentiality concern. J Adolesc Health. 2007;40(3):218–26.

88. Reddy DM, Fleming R, Swain C. Effect of mandatory parental notification on adolescent girls' use of sexual health care services. JAMA. 2002;288(6):710–4.

89. International Covenant on Civil and Political Rights. New York (NY): United Nations; 1966.

90. Cook RJ, Dickens BM. Considerations for formulating reproductive health laws, 2nd edition. Geneva: World Health Organization; 2000.

91. Interagency statement on forced or coerced sterilization. Geneva: World Health Organization; 2014.

92. Views on Communication 4/2004: Ms. A. S. v. Hungary. New York (NY): United Nations Committee on the Elimination of Discrimination against Women; 2006 (CEDAW/C/36/D/4/2004).

93. Report of the Special Rapporteur on the right of everyone to the enjoyment of the highest attainable standard of physical and mental health, Anand Grover. New York (NY): United Nations; 2009.

94. Eliminating female genital mutilation: an interagency statement. Geneva: World Health Organization; 2008.

95. Nour NM, Michels KB, Bryant AE. Defibulation to treat female genital cutting: effect on symptoms and sexual function. Obstet Gynecol. 2006;108(1):55–60.

96. Effects of female genital mutilation on childbirth in Africa. Policy Brief. Geneva: World Health Organization; 2008.

97. Global strategy to stop health-care providers from performing female genital mutilation. Geneva: World Health Organization; 2011.

98. Standards of care for the health of transsexual, transgender, and gender nonconforming people, 7th version. World Professional Association for Transgender Health (WPATH); 2012 (http://www.wpath.org/site_page.cfm?pk_association_webpage_menu=1351&pk_association_webpage=3926http://www.wpath.org/, accessed 22 January 2015).

99. World report on disability. Geneva: World Health Organization; 2011.

100. Cottingham J, Berer M. Access to essential medicines for sexual and reproductive health care: the role of the pharmaceutical industry and international regulation. Reprod Health Matters. 2011;19(38):69–84.

101. World Health Assembly discusses the issue of quality medicines. Brussels: Reproductive Health Supplies Coalition; 2011 (http://www.rhsupplies.org/nc/sp/news/newsview/article/world-health-assembly-discusses-the-issue-of-quality-medicines.html, accessed 5 February 2015).

102. Fake antibiotics found in six states. Partnership for Safe Medicines; 2011 (http://www.safemedicines.org/2011/05/fake-antibiotics-found-in-six-states-246.html, accessed 5 February 2015).

103. Closing the gap in a generation: health equity through action on the social determinants of health. Final report of the Commission on the Social Determinants of Health. Geneva: World Health Organization; 2008.

104. Reza-Paul S, Beattie T, Syed HUR, et al. Declines in risk behaviour and sexually transmitted infection prevalence following a community-led HIV preventive intervention among female sex workers in Mysore, India. AIDS. 2008;22 (Supplement 5):S91–S100.

105. Ramesh BM, Beattie TSH, Shajy I, et al. Changes in risk behaviours and prevalence of sexually transmitted infections following HIV preventive interventions among female sex workers in five districts in Karnataka state, south India. Sex Transm Infect. 2010;86 (Supplement 1):117–24.

106. Foss AM, Hossain M, Vickerman PT, et al. A systematic review of published evidence on intervention impact on condom use in sub-Saharan Africa and Asia. Sex Transm Infect. 2007;83(7):510-516.

107. General Comment No. 20: Non-discrimination in economic, social and cultural rights (art. 2, para. 2, of the International Covenant on Economic, Social and Cultural Rights). New York (NY): United Nations Committee on Economic, Social and Cultural Rights; 2009 (E/C.12/GC/20).

108. Views on Communication No. 488/1992: Toonen v. Australia. Geneva: United Nations Human Rights Committee; 1994 (CCPR/C/50/D/488/1992).

109. Law No. 38 of 2005: Children's Act, 2005, amended by No. 41 of 2007: Children's Amendment Act, 2007. Section 134. Republic of South Africa; 2005.

110. General Recommendation No. 21: Equality in marriage and family relations. New York (NY): United Nations Committee on the Elimination of Discrimination against Women; 1994 (A/49/38).

111. How to get to zero: faster, smarter, better. World AIDS day report. Geneva: Joint United Nations Programme on HIV/AIDS (UNAIDS); 2011.

112. Joint Statement by the United Nations Working Group on discrimination against women in law and in practice: Adultery as a criminal offence violates women's human rights. Geneva: United Nations Office of the High Commissioner for Human Rights; 2012.

113. Wijesundera v. Wijekoon. C.A. 15/86, decided on 5 and 6 June 1990. Democratic Socialist Republic of Sri Lanka Court of Appeal; 1990.

114. Report of the Committee on the Elimination of Discrimination against Women. Twenty-fourth and twenty-fifth session. New York (NY): United Nations; 2001 (A/56/38 (Supp) Chapter IV. Consideration of reports submitted by States Parties under article 18 of the Convention. Section B.1. Initial periodic report of Burundi and Section B.5. Third and combined fourth and fifth periodic reports of Egypt).

115. Guidelines on international protection: gender-related persecution within the context of Article 1A(2) of the 1951 Convention and/or its 1967 Protocol relating to the Status of Refugees. Geneva: United Nations High Commissioner for Refugees; 2002.

116. Law 24.453 of 1995. Argentina; 2005.

117. Law 11.106. Brazil; 2005.

118. *Expediente 936-95*, decided on 7 March 1996. República de Guatemala Corte de Constitucionalidad [Guatemala Constitutional Court]; 1996 (in Spanish).

119. Karner v. Austria. Application No. 40016/98. Strasbourg: European Court of Human Rights; 2003.

120. Views on Communication No. 941/2000: Young v. Australia. Geneva: United Nations Human Rights Committee (CCPR/C/78/D941/2000).

121. Discriminatory laws and practices and acts of violence against individuals based on their sexual orientation and gender identity. Report of the United Nations High Commissioner for Human Rights. New York (NY): United Nations General Assembly; 2011.

122. Discrimination on the basis of sexual orientation and gender identity (Doc. 12087). Strasbourg; Council of Europe, Parliamentary Assembly; 2009.

123. El Al Israel Airlines Ltd. v. Yonatan Danilowitz. Case No. 721/94, decided on 30 November 1994. Israel Supreme Court; 1994.

124. Justiça Federal da República Federativa do Brasil. *Resolução No. 175 de 14 de maio de 2013* [Resolution No. 175 of 14 May 2013]. Brasília: Conselho Nacional de Justiça; 2013 (in Portuguese).

125. Public Act 1993 No. 82: Human Right Act 1993. New Zealand; 1993.

126. Public Act 2004 No. 102: Civil Union Act 2004. New Zealand; 2004.

127. Decision U-I-425/06-10 of 2 July 2009. Republic of Slovenia Constitutional Court; 2009.

128. *Boletin Oficial de la República Argentina Buenos Aires, jueves 22 de julio de 2010* [Official Bulletin of the Republic of Argentina, Buenos Aires, Thursday 22 July 2010]. Buenos Aires: República Argentina; 2010 (in Spanish).

129. Minister of Home Affairs and Another v. Fourie and Another (CCT 60/04) [2005] ZACC 19. Constitutional Court of South Africa; 2005.

130. *Wet van 21 december 2000 tot wijziging van Boek 1 van het Burgerlijk Wetboek in verband met de openstelling van het huwelijk voor personen van hetzelfde geslacht (Wet openstelling huwelijk)* [Law of 21 December 2000 amending Book 1 of the Dutch Civil Code in connection with the opening of marriage to same-sex couples (Act opening marriage)]. The Netherlands: Staatsblad van het Koninkrijk der Nederlanden; 2001 (in Dutch).

131. *LOI n° 2013-404 du 17 mai 2013 ouvrant le mariage aux couples de personnes de même sexe.* NOR: JUSC1236338L [Law No. 2013-404 of 17 May 2013 opening marriage to same-sex couples]. France; 2013 (in French) (http://www.legifrance.gouv.fr/eli/loi/2013/5/17/ JUSC1236338L/jo/texte, accessed 5 May 2014).

132. Halpern et al. v. Attorney General of Canada (2003) O.J. No. 2268. Toronto: Court of Appeal for Ontario; 2003.

133. Public Act 2013 No. 20: Marriage (Definition of Marriage) Amendment Act 2013. Date of assent 19 April 2013. New Zealand; 2013.

134. Small W, Wood E, Betteridge G, Montaner J, Kerr T. The impact of incarceration upon adherence to HIV treatment among HIV-positive injection drug users: a qualitative study. AIDS Care. 2009;21(6):708–14.

135. Maruschak LM. HIV in prisons and jails 1999. NCJ 187456. Washington (DC): Bureau of Justice Statistics Bulletin; 2001.

136. Maruschak LM. HIV in prisons, 2006. Statistical tables, NCJ 222179. Washington (DC): Bureau of Justice Statistics; 2008.

137. Clarke JG, Hebert MR, Rosengard C, Rose JS, DaSilva KM, Stein MD. Reproductive health care and family planning needs among incarcerated women. Am J Public Health. 2006;96(5):834–9.

138. Standard Minimum Rules for the Treatment of Prisoners. New York (NY): United Nations; 1977.

139. Code of Conduct for Law Enforcement Officials. New York (NY): United Nations; 1979.

140. United Nations Standard Minimum Rules for the Administration of Juvenile Justice ("The Beijing Rules"). New York (NY): United Nations; 1985.

141. Body of Principles for the Protection of All Persons under Any Form of Detention or Imprisonment. New York (NY): United Nations; 1988 (Principles 24 and 25).

142. Basic Principles for the Treatment of Prisoners. New York (NY): United Nations; 1990.

143. United Nations Rules for the Protection of Juveniles Deprived of their Liberty. New York (NY): United Nations; 1990.

144. General Comment No. 15: The position of aliens under the Covenant. Geneva: United Nations Human Rights Committee; 1986 (HRI/GEN/1/Rev.1 at 18 (1994)).

145. "Will I have to pay?" London: National AIDS Trust; 2007 (http://www.nat.org.uk/Media%20library/Files/PDF%20documents/2009/Feb/Will%20I%20Have%20to%20Pay%20April%202007-1.pdf, accessed 5 February 2015).

146. United Nations High Commissioner for Refugees (UNHCR), World Health Organization and Joint United Nations Programme on HIV/AIDS. Policy statement on HIV testing and counselling in health facilities for refugees, internally displaced persons and other persons of concern to UNHCR. Geneva: UNHCR; 2009.

147. UNAIDS report on the global AIDS epidemic 2010. Geneva: Joint United Nations Programme on HIV/AIDS (UNAIDS); 2010.

148. Burris S, Cameron E. The case against criminalization of HIV transmission. JAMA. 2008;300(5):578–81.

149. Cameron E, Burris S, Clayton M. HIV is a virus, not a crime. HIV/AIDS Policy & Law Review/Canadian HIV/AIDS Legal Network. 2008;13(2-3):64–8.

150. Joint United Nations Programme on HIV/AIDS (UNAIDS), United Nations Development Programme. Policy Brief: Criminalization of HIV transmission. Geneva: UNAIDS; 2008.

151. Wingwood GM, DiClemente RJ, Mikhail I, McCree DH, Davies SL, Hardin JW, et al. HIV discrimination and the health of women living with HIV. Women and Health. 2007;46(2-3):99–112.

152. Kinsler JJ, Wong MD, Sayles JN, et al. The effect of perceived stigma from a health care provider on access to care among a low-income HIV-positive population. AIDS Patient Care STDs. 2007;21(8):584–92.

153. Sayles JN, Wong MD, Kinsler JJ, Martins D, Cunningham WE. The association of stigma with self-reported access to medical care and antiretroviral therapy adherence in persons living with HIV/AIDS. J Gen Intern Med. 2009;24(10):1101–8.

154. Wang Y, Zhang KN, Zhang KL. HIV/AIDS related discrimination in health care service: a cross-sectional study in Gejiu City, Yunan Province. Biomed Environ Sci. 2008;21(2):124–8.

155. Ahmed A, Kaplan M, Symington A, Kismödi E. Criminalising consensual sexual behaviour in the context of HIV: consequences, evidence, and leadership. Glob Public Health. 2011;6(Suppl 3):S357–69.

156. Mr S v. Mr S2 and Ms R, Order of Geneva Court of Justice, decided on 23 February 2009. Geneva: Geneva Court of Justice; 2009.

157. CRI-2004-085-009168. New Zealand: District Court Wellington; 2005.

158. Vernazza P, Hirschel B, Bernasconi E, Flepp M. *Les personnes séropositives ne souffrant d'aucune autre MST et suivant un traitement antirétroviral efficace ne transmettent pas le VIH par voie sexuelle* [People not suffering from another STI and who are following an effective antiretroviral treatment do not sexually transmit HIV]. Bulletin des Médecins Suisses. 2008;89:5 (in French).

159. Wolf L, Vezina R. Crime and punishment: Is there a role for criminal law in HIV prevention policy? Whittier Law Rev. 2004;(25):821–86.

160. Dodds C, Weatherburn P, Bourne A, Hammond G, Weait M, Hickson F, et al. Sexually charged: the views of gay and bisexual men on criminal prosecutions for sexual HIV transmission. London: Sigma Research; 2009.

161. Grierson J, Power J, Croy S, Clement T, Thorpe R, McDonald K, et al. HIV Futures 6: Making positive lives count. The Living with HIV Program. Melbourne: Australian Research Centre in Sex, Health and Society, La Trobe University; 2006.

162. Ten reasons to oppose the criminalization of HIV exposure or transmission. New York (NY): Open Society Institute; 2008.

163. Gielen AC, McDonnell KA, Burke JG, O'Campo P. Women's lives after an HIV positive diagnosis: disclosure and violence. Matern Child Health J. 2000;4(2):111–20.

164. AIDS discrimination in Asia. Global Network of People Living with HIV; 2004 (http://www.gnpplus.net/resources/aids-discrimination-in-asia/, accessed 1 May 2014).

165. First Global Parliamentary Meeting on HIV/AIDS, Manila, Philippines, 28–30 November 2007. Final Conclusions. Geneva: Inter-Parliamentary Union; 2007.

166. Ending overly broad criminalization of HIV non-disclosure, exposure and transmission: critical scientific, medical and legal considerations. Guidance Note. Geneva: Joint United Nations Programme on HIV/AIDS (UNAIDS); 2013.

167. Republic Act 8504: The Philippine AIDS Prevention and Control Act of 1998. Republic of the Philippines; 1998.

168. International guidelines on HIV/AIDS and human rights – 2006 consolidated version. Geneva: Joint United Nations Programme on HIV/AIDS (UNAIDS) and the Office of the United Nations High Commissioner for Human Rights (OHCHR); 2006.

169. General Comment No. 5: Persons with disabilities. New York (NY): United Nations Committee on Economic, Social and Cultural Rights; 1994 (E/1995/22).

170. Prevention and treatment of HIV and other sexually transmitted infections for sex workers in low- and middle-income countries. Geneva: World Health Organization; 2012.

171. Rutledge SE, Abell N, Padmore J, McCan TJ. AIDS stigma in health services in the Eastern Caribbean. Sociol Health Illn. 2009;31(1):17–34.

172. Johnson CA. Off the map: how HIV/AIDS programming is failing same-sex practicing people in Africa. New York (NY): International Gay and Lesbian Human Rights Commission; 2007.

173. Niang CI, Diagne M, Niang Y, Moreau AM, Gomis D, Diouf M, et al. Meeting the sexual health needs of men who have sex with men in Senegal. New York (NY): Population Council; 2002.

174. Wells H, Polders L. Gay and lesbian people's experience of the health care sector in Guateng. Arcadia, South Africa: OUT LGBT Well-being; 2007.

175. Discrimination on grounds of sexual orientation and gender identity in Europe, 2nd edition. Strasbourg: Council of Europe; 2011.

176. European Commission Directorate-General for Justice. Trans and intersex people – discrimination on the grounds of sex, gender identity, and gender expression. Luxembourg: Office for Official Publications of the European Union; 2012.

177. Trans people across the world face substantial barriers to adequate health and health care. New York (NY): Open Society Foundations; 2013.

178. Report of the Special Rapporteur on torture and other cruel, inhuman or degrading treatment or punishment, Juan E. Méndez. New York (NY): United Nations General Assembly; 2013.

179. Concluding observations: Combined fourth, fifth, sixth and seventh periodic reports: Uganda. New York (NY): United Nations Committee on the Elimination of Discrimination against Women; 2010 (CEDAW/C/UGA/CO/7).

180. Recommendation 1474 (2000) on the situation of lesbians and gays in Council of Europe Member States. Strasbourg: Council of Europe, Parliamentary Assembly; 2000.

181. Resolution of 26 April 2007 on homophobia in Europe. P6_TA(2007)0167. European Parliament; 2007.

182. *Caso Atala Riffo y niñas v. Chile (Fondo, reparaciones y costas)*, decided on 24 February 2012. San José, Costa Rica: Inter-American Court of Human Rights; 2012.

183. General Assembly Resolution: Human rights, sexual orientation and gender identity. 3 June 2008. Washington (DC): Organization of American States; 2008 (OAS/AG/RES.2435 (XXXVIII-O/08)).

184. General Assembly Resolution: Human rights, sexual orientation and gender identity. 4 June 2009. Washington (DC): Organization of American States; 2009 (OAS/AG/RES.2504 (XXXIX-O/09)).

185. Human rights, sexual orientation and gender identity. Resolution adopted 15 June 2011. New York (NY): United Nations General Assembly; 2011.

186. Recommendation CM/REC(2010)5 on measures to combat discrimination on grounds of sexual orientation or gender identity. Strasbourg: Council of Europe, Committee of Ministers; 2010.

187. Recommendation 924 (1981) on discrimination against homosexuals. Strasbourg: Council of Europe, Parliamentary Assembly; 1981.

188. Dudgeon v. the United Kingdom. Application No. 7525/76, decided on 22 October 1981. Strasbourg: European Court of Human Rights; 1981.

189. Concluding observations of the Human Rights Committee: Chile. Fifth periodic report. Geneva: United Nations Human Rights Committee; 2007 (CCPR/C/CHL/CO/5).

190. Concluding observations of the Human Rights Committee: Uzbekistan. Third periodic report. Geneva: United Nations Human Rights Committee; 2008 (CCPR/C/UZB/CO/3).

191. Concluding observations of the Human Rights Committee: Grenada. New York (NY): United Nations Human Rights Committee; 2010 (CCPR/C/GRD/CO/1).

192. Concluding observations of the Human Rights Committee: El Salvador. Sixth periodic report. Geneva: United Nations Human Rights Committee; 2010 (CCPR/C/SLV/CO/6).

193. Concluding observations of the Human Rights Committee: Togo. Fourth periodic report. Geneva: United Nations Human Rights Committee; 2011 (CCPR/C/TGO/CO/4).

194. National Coalition for Gay and Lesbian Equality and Another v. Minister of Justice and Others. Case CCT 11/98, decided 9 October 1998. Republic of South Africa, Constitutional Court; 1998.

195. *Decreto 100 de 1980: Por el cual se expide el nuevo Código Penal, el 23 de enero 1980.* [Decree 100 of 1980 whereby the new Penal Code is issued, 23 January 1980]. República de Colombia; 1980 (in Spanish).

196. *Ley 1047*, 23 December 1998. República de Chile; 1998 (in Spanish).

197. *Código penal, Ley No. 641, 5 mayo 2008.* [Penal Code, Law No. 641, 5 May 2008]. República de Nicaragua; 2008 (in Spanish).

198. Crimes Decree 2009 (Decree No. 44 of 2009). Republic of Fiji; 2009.

199. Constitution of the Republic of South Africa. Republic of South Africa; 1996.

200. Hill DB. Genderism, transphobia, and gender bashing: A framework for interpreting anti-transgender violence. In: Wallace B, Carter R, editors. A multicultural approach for understanding and dealing with violence: a handbook for psychologists and educators. Thousand Oaks (CA): Sage Publishing; 2001.

201. United Nations Development Programme. Discussion paper: Transgender health and human rights. New York (NY): United Nations Development Programme; 2013.

202. Grossman AH, D'Augelli AR, Salter NP. Male-to-female transgender youth: gender expression milestones, gender atypicality, victimization, and parents' responses. J GLBT Fam Stud. 2006;2(1):71–92.

203. Sugano E, Nemoto T, Operario D. The impact of exposure to transphobia on HIV risk behavior in a sample of transgendered women of color in San Francisco. AIDS Behav. 2006;10(2):217–25.

204. Castagnoli C. Transgender persons' rights in the EU Member States. Brussels: Directorate General for Internal Policies, Citizens' Rights and Constitutional Affairs, Civil Liberties, Justice and Home Affairs, European Parliament; 2010.

205. Eliason MJ, Hughes T. Treatment counselor's attitudes about lesbian, gay, and transgendered clients: urban vs rural settings. Subst Use Misuse. 2004;39(4):625–44.

206. Guevara AL. The hidden HIV epidemic: transgender women in Latin America and Asia, compilation of epidemiological data. Buenos Aires: International HIV/AIDS Alliance; 2009.

207. Ojanen T. Sexual/gender minorities in Thailand: identities, challenges and voluntary-sector counselling. Sex Res Soc Policy. 2009;6(2):4–34.

208. Sood N. Transgender people's access to sexual health and rights: a study of law and policy in 12 Asian countries. Kuala Lumpur: Asian-Pacific Resource and Research Centre for Women (ARROW); 2009.

209. Best practices guide to trans health care in the national health system. Spanish Network for Depathologization of Trans Identities; 2010.

210. Transforming health. International rights based advocacy for trans health. New York (NY): Open Society Foundations; 2013.

211. Transgender Health Program guidelines for transgender care. Vancouver Coastal Health; 2012 (http://transhealth.vch.ca/resources/careguidelines.html, accessed 5 May 2014).

212. Ainsworth TA, Spiegel JH. Quality of life of individuals with and without facial feminization surgery or gender reassignment surgery. Qual Life Res. 2010;19(7):1019–24.

213. De Cuypere G, T'Sjoen G, Beerten R, Selvaggi G, De Sutter P, Hoebeke P, et al. Sexual and physical health after sex reassignment surgery. Arch Sex Behav. 2005;34(6):679–90.

214. Hembree W, Cohen-Kettenis P, Delemarre-van de Waal HA, Gooren LJ, Meyer 3rd WJ, Spack NP, et al. Endocrine treatment of transsexual persons: an Endocrine Society clinical practice guideline. J Clin Endocrinol Metab. 2009;94(9):3132–54.

215. Monstrey S, Ceulemans P, Hoebeke P. Sex reassignment surgery in the female-to-male transsexual. Semin Plast Surg. 2011;25(3):229–44.

216. Pfäfflin F, Junge A. Sex reassignment. Thirty years of international follow-up studies after sex reassignment surgery: a comprehensive review, 1961–1991. Dusseldorf: Symposium Publishing; 1998 [Translated from German into American English by Roberta B. Jacobson and Alf B. Meier] (http://www.symposion.com/ijt/pfaefflin/1000.htm, accessed 10 January 2015).

217. Selvaggi G, Monstrey S, Ceulemans P, T'Sjoen G, De Cuypere G, Hoebeke P. Genital sensitivity after sex reassignment surgery in transsexual patients. Ann Plast Surg. 2007;58(4):427–33.

218. Weyers S, Elaut E, De Sutter P, Gerris J, T'Sjoen G, Heylens G, et al. Long-term assessment of the physical, mental and sexual health among transsexual women. Sex Med. 2009;6(3):752–60.

219. Clarification on medical necessity of treatment, sex reassignment, and insurance coverage in the USA. World Professional Association for Transgender Health (WPATH); 2008.

220. Lobato et al. 2005. Cited in: Todahl JL, Linviole D, Bustin A, Wheeler J, Gau J. Sexual assault support services and community systems: understanding critical issues and needs in the LGBTQ community. J Violence Against Women. 2009;15(8):952–76. doi:10.1177/1077801209335494.

221. Bockting WO, Robinson BE, Rosser BRS. Transgender HIV prevention: a qualitative needs assessment. AIDS Care. 1998;10:505–26.

222. Lombardi EL, van Servellen G. Building culturally sensitive substance use prevention and treatment programs for transgendered populations. J Subst Abuse Treat. 2000;19:291–6.

223. Lombardi E. Enhancing transgender health care. Am J Public Health. 2001;91:869–72.

224. Cohen-Kettenis PT, Delemarre-van der Waal H, Gooren LJG. The treatment of adolescent transsexuals: changing insights. J Sex Med. 2008;5:1892–7.

225. Giordano S. Lives in a chiaroscuro. Should we suspend the puberty of children with gender identity disorder? J Med Ethics. 2008;34(8):580–4.

226. Nuttbrock L, Hwahng S, Bockting W, Rosenblum A, Mason M, Macri M, Becker J. Psychiatric impact of gender-related abuse across the life course of male-to-female transgender persons. J Sex Res. 2010;47(1):12–23.

227. Cameron L. Sex workers, transgender people and men who have sex with men: Thailand. New York (NY): Open Society Institute, Sexual Health and Rights program; 2006.

228. Clements-Nolle K, Marx R, Guzman R, Katz M. HIV prevalence, risk behaviors, health care use, and mental health status of transgender persons: implications for public health intervention. Am J Public Health. 2001;91(6):915–21.

229. Grossman AH, D'Augelli AR. Transgender youth: invisible and vulnerable. J Homosex. 2006;51(1):111–28.

230. McGowan K. Transgender needs assessment. New York (NY): The HIV Prevention Planning Unit of the New York City Department of Health; 1999.

231. Sanchez NF, Sanchez JP, Danoff A. Health care utilization, barriers to care, and hormone usage among male-to-female transgender persons in New York City. Am J Public Health. 2009;99(4):713–9.

232. Teh YK. *Mak nyahs* (male transsexuals) in Malaysia: the influence of culture and religion on their Identity. Int J Transgenderism. 2001;5(3).

233. Winter S. Thai transgenders in focus: demographics, transitions and identities. Int J Transgenderism. 2006;9(1):15–27.

234. Xavier JM, Simmons R. The Washington Transgender Needs Assessment Survey. Washington (DC): US Helping Us – People Into Living, Inc., and the Administration for HIV/AIDS, Department of Health, District of Columbia; 2000 (http://www.glaa.org/archive/2000/tgneedsassessment1112.shtml, accessed 5 February 2015).

235. Coleman E, Bockting W, Botzer M, Cohen-Kettenis P, DeCuypere G, Feldman J, et al. Standards of care for the health of transsexual, transgender, and gender-nonconforming people, version 7. Int J Transgenderism. 2011;13(4):165–232. doi:10.1080/15532739.2011.700873.

236. Shumer DE, Spack NP. Current management of gender identity disorder in childhood and adolescence: guidelines, barriers and areas of controversy. Curr Opin Endocrinol Diabetes Obes. 2013;20(1):69–73.

237. Bockting WO, Robinson BE, Forberg J, Scheltema K. Evaluation of a sexual health approach to reducing HIV/STD risk in the transgender community. AIDS Care. 2005;17(3):289–303.

238. McGovern SJ. Self-castration in a transsexual. J Accid Emerg Med.1995;12(1):57–8.

239. Sex reassignment surgery (SRS): backgrounder. In: Egale Canada Human Rights Trust [website]. Toronto: Egale Canada Human Rights Trust; 2004 (http://egale.ca/all/sex-reassignment-surgery-srs-backgrounder/, accessed 5 February 2015).

240. Landén M, Wålinder J, Hambert G, Lundström B. Factors predictive of regret in sex reassignment. Acta Psychiatr Scand. 1998;97(4):284–9.

241. Position statement on access to care for transgender and gender variant individuals. American Psychiatric Association; 2012 (http://www.psychiatry.org/File%20Library/Advocacy%20and%20Newsroom/Position%20Statements/ps2012_TransgenderCare.pdf, accessed 5 February 2015).

242. General Recommendation 28: Core obligations of States Parties under Article 2 of the Convention of the Elimination of All Forms of Discrimination against Women. New York (NY): United Nations Committee on the Elimination of Discrimination against Women; 2010 (CEDAW/C/20107477GC.2).

243. Resolution on transgender and gender identity and gender expression non-discrimination. American Psychological Association; 2008 (www.apa.org/about/policy/chapter-12b.aspx#transgender, accessed 5 February 2015).

244. Van Kück v. Germany. Application No. 35968/97, decided on 12 June 2003. Strasbourg: European Court of Human Rights; 2003.

245. *Ley 26743: Derecho a la identidad de género.* [Law No. 26743: Right to gender identity]. República Argentina; 2012 (in Spanish).

246. Köhler R, Richer A, Ehrt J. Legal gender recognition in Europe: toolkit. Transgender Europe; 2013 (http://www.tgeu.org/sites/default/files/Toolkit_web.pdf, accessed 5 January 2015).

247. B v. France. Application No. 13343/87, decided on 25 March 1992. Strasbourg: European Court of Human Rights; 1992.

248. Goodwin v. United Kingdom. Application No. 28957/95, decided on 11 July 2002. Strasbourg: European Court of Human Rights; 2002.

249. Decision T-594/93, decided 15 December 1993. Constitutional Court of Colombia; 1993.

250. Concluding observations: Ireland. Geneva: United Nations Human Rights Committee; 2008 (CCPR/C/IRL/CO/3).

251. Concluding observations: United Kingdom of Great Britain and Northern Ireland. Geneva: United Nations Human Rights Committee; 2008 (CCPR/C/GBR/6).

252. VwGH 27.02.2009, 2008/17/0054, decided 27 February 2009. Austrian Administrative High Court; 2009.

253. 1 BvL 10/05. (27 May 2008). Federal Constitutional Court of Germany; 2008.

254. 1 BvR 3295/07. (11 January 2011). Federal Constitutional Court of Germany; 2011.

255. Decision No. 161 of 1985. Italian Constitutional Court; 1985.

256. Michael v. Registrar-General of Births, Deaths and Marriages, 9 June 2008. New Zealand Family Court; 2008 (FAM-2006-004-002325).

257. *Lov om ændring af lov om Det Centrale Personregister.* 2014 LOV nr 752 af 25/06/2014 [Law amending the law on the central registry of persons]. Denmark: Økonomi-og Indenrigsministeriet; 2014 (in Danish).

258. Gender Identity Act. 30/10/2014. Malta; 2014.

259. Sexual orientation, gender identity and justice: a comparative law casebook. Geneva: International Commission of Jurists; 2011.

260. Supreme Court of Nepal. Sunil Babu Pant and others v. Government of Nepal and others. Writ No. 917, 21 December 2007 [English translation]. NJA Law Journal. 2008:261–86.

261. Dr. Mohammad Aslam Khaki and Anr. V. Senior Superintendent of Police (Operation) Rawalpindi and Ors. Constitution Petition No. 43 of 2009, decided on 22 March 2011. Supreme Court of Pakistan; 2011.

262. Karkazis K. Fixing sex: intersex, medical authority, and lived experience. Durham (NC): Duke University Press; 2008.

263. Parens E, editor. Surgically shaping children: technology, ethics and the pursuit of normality. Baltimore (MA): Johns Hopkins University Press; 2006.

264. Concluding observations: Germany. Geneva: United Nations Committee against Torture; 2011 (CAT/C/DEU/CO/5).

265. Cools M et al. Germ cell tumors in the intersex gonad: old paths, new directions, moving frontiers. Endocr Rev. 2006;27(5):S468–484.

266. Crouch NS, Creighton SM. Long-term functional outcomes in female genital reconstruction in childhood. BJU Int. 2007;100:403.

267. Goran LJ, Giltay EJ, Bunck MC. Long-term treatment of transsexuals with cross-sex hormones: extensive personal experience. J Clin Endocrinol Metab. 2008;93(1):19–25.

268. Shifting the paradigm of intersex treatment. Rohnert Park (CA): Intersex Society of North America; Undated (http://www.isna.org/compare, accessed 5 February 2015).

269. Karkazis K, Rossi W. Disorder of sex development: optimizing care. Pediatr Rev. 2010;31;e82–e85.

270. Tamar-Mattis A. Sterilization and minors with intersex conditions in California law. California Law Review Circuit. 2012;3(1):126–35.

271. Intersexualität. Stellungnahme des Deutschen Ethikrats. Berlin: Deutscher Ethikrat; 2012.

272. Discriminatory laws and practices and acts of violence against individuals based on their sexual orientation and gender identity. Report of the United Nations High Commissioner for Human Rights. New York (NY): United Nations General Assembly; 2011 (A/HRC/19/41).

273. Wisniewski A, Mazur T. 46,XY DSD with female or ambiguous external genitalia at birth due to Androgen Insensitivity Syndrome, 5-Reductase-2 Deficiency, or 17-Hydroxysteroid Dehydrogenase Deficiency: a review of quality of life outcomes. Int J Pediatr Endocrinol. 2009;567430.

274. Murphy C, Allen L, Jamieson MA. Ambiguous genitalia in the newborn: an overview and teaching tool. J Pediatr Adolesc Gynecol. 2011;24(5):236–50.

275. On the management of differences of sex development: ethical issues relating to "intersexuality". Berne: Swiss National Advisory Commission on Biomedical Ethics NEK-CNE; 2012 (Opinion 20/2012).

276. Intersex: treatment (updated 14 April 2014). In: University of Maryland Medical Center [website]. Baltimore (MD): University of Maryland Medical Center; 2014 (http://www.umm.edu/ency/article/001669trt.htm, accessed 4 February 2015).

277. Betteridge G. Sex, work, rights: reforming Canadian criminal laws on prostitution. Toronto: Canadian HIV/AIDS Legal Network; 2005.

278. Day SE, Ward H. British policy makes sex workers vulnerable. BMJ. 2007;334(7586):187. doi:10.1136/bmj.39104.638785.59.

279. Reckart ML Sex-work harm reduction. Lancet. 2005;366:2123–34.

280. UNAIDS Guidance note on HIV and sex work. Geneva: Joint United Nations Programme on HIV/AIDS (UNAIDS); 2009.

281. Burris S, Overs C, Weait M. Laws and practices that effectively criminalise people living with HIV and vulnerable to HIV. Paper prepared for First Meeting of the Global Commission on HIV and the Law, 6–7 October 2010, New York (NY).

282. Mossman E. International approaches to decriminalising or legalising prostitution. Wellington, New Zealand: Ministry of Justice; 2007.

283. The report of the UNAIDS Advisory Group on HIV and sex work. Geneva: Joint United Nations Programme on HIV/AIDS (UNAIDS); 2011.

284. Benoit C, Millar A. Dispelling myths and understanding realities: working conditions, health status and exiting experiences of sex workers. British Columbia, Canada: Prostitutes Empowerment, Education and Resource Society; 2001.

285. Shannon K, Rusch M, Shoveller J, Alexson D, Gibson K, Tyndall MW; Maka Project Partnership. Mapping violence and policing as an environmental – structural barrier to health service and syringe availability among substance-using women in street-level sex work. Int J Drug Policy. 2008;19(2):140–7.

286. Tucker JD, Ren X. Sex worker incarcerations in the People's Republic of China. Sex Transm Infect. 2008;84:34–5. doi:10.1136/sti.2007.027235.

287. United Nations Population Fund (UNFPA) Namibia, Joint United Nations Programme on HIV/AIDS (UNAIDS) Namibia. Sex work, HIV and access to health services in Namibia: national meeting report and recommendations. Windhoek: UNFPA/Namibia; 2011.

288. Ghimire L, van Teijlingen E. Barriers to utilisation of sexual health services by female sex workers in Nepal. Glob J Health Sci. 2009;1(1):12–22.

289. Pauw L, Brenner L. "You are just whores – you can't be raped": barriers to safer sex practices among women street sex workers in Cape Town. Cult Health Sex. 2003;5(6):465–81.

290. Eight working papers/case studies: examining the intersections of sex work law, policy, rights and health. New York (NY): Open Society Institute; 2006.

291. Simsek S, Kisa A, Dziegelewski SF. Sex workers and the issues surrounding registration in Turkey. J Health Soc Policy. 2003;17(3):55–69.

292. General Recommendation No. 19: Violence against women. New York (NY): United Nations Committee on the Elimination of Discrimination against Women; 1992 (A/47/38).

293. Optional Protocol to the Convention on the Rights of the Child on the sale of children, child prostitution and child pornography. New York (NY): United Nations Committee on the Rights of the Child; 2000 (A/RES/54/263; entered into force 18 January 2002).

294. Brothels Task Force. Report of the Brothels Task Force. Sydney: New South Wales Government; 2001.

295. Prostitution Control Regulations 2006, S.R. No. 64/2006. State of Victoria, Commonwealth of Australia; 2006.

296. O'Connor CC, Berry G, Rohrsheim R, Donovan B. Sexual health and the use of condoms among local and international sex workers in Sydney. Genitourin Med. 1996;72:47–51.

297. Pyett PM, Haste BR, Snow J. Risk practices for HIV infection and other STDs among female prostitutes working in legalized brothels. AIDS Care. 1996;8(1):85–94.

298. Dutch Policy on Prostitution. Questions and answers 2012. Dutch Ministry of Foreign Affairs; 2012 (http://www.minbuza.nl/binaries/content/assets/minbuza/en/import/en/you_and_the_netherlands/about_the_netherlands/ethical_issues/faq-prostitutie-pdf--engels.pdf-2012.pdf, accessed 5 May 2014).

299. Prostitution Reform Act 2003. Public Act 2003 No. 28. New Zealand; 2003.

300. Sentencia T-629/10, decided on 13 August 2010. República de Colombia Corte Constitucional [Constitutional Court of the Republic of Colombia]; 2010 (in Spanish).

301. Kylie v. Commission for Conciliation Mediation and Arbitration and Others. Case No. CA10/08, decided on 26 May 2010. South Africa Labour Appeals Court; 2010.

302. Bangladesh Society for the Enforcement of Human Rights and Others v. Government of Bangladesh and Others. Case 53 DLR (2001) 1. Dhaka: High Court Division, Bangladesh Supreme Court; 2000.

303. Convention 182: Worst forms of child labour. Geneva: International Labour Organization; 1999.

304. Profiting from abuse. An investigation into the sexual exploitation of our children. New York (NY): United Nations Children's Fund; 2001.

305. International technical guidance on sexuality education. Paris: United Nations Educational, Scientific and Cultural Organization; 2009.

306. Kirby D. The impact of schools and school programs on adolescent sexual behaviour. J Sex Res. 2002;39(1):2733.

307. Kirby D. Sex and HIV programs: their impact on sexual behaviors of young people throughout the world. J Adolesc Health. 2007;40:206–17.

308. Lazarus JV, Sihvonen-Riemenschneider H, Laukamm-Josten U, Wong F, Liljestrand J. Systematic review of interventions to prevent the spread of sexually transmitted infections, including HIV, among young people in Europe. Croat Med J. 2010;51(1):74–84.

309. Michielsen K, Chersich MF, Luchters S, De Koker P, Van Rossem R, Temmerman M. Effectiveness of HIV prevention for youth in sub-Saharan Africa: systematic review and meta-analysis of randomized and nonrandomized trials. AIDS. 2010;24(8):1193–202.

310. Oringanje C, Meremikwu MM, Eko H, Esu E, Meremikwu A, Ehiri JE. Interventions for preventing unintended pregnancies among adolescents. Cochrane Database Syst Rev. 2009;4. doi:10.1002/14651858.CD005215.pub2.

311. Robin L, Dittus P, Whitaker D, Crosby R, Ethier K, Mezoff J, et al. Behavioral interventions to reduce incidence of HIV, STD, and pregnancy among adolescents: a decade in review. J Adol Health. 2004;34(1):3–26.

312. Morris R. Research and evaluation in sexuality education: an allegorical exploration of complexities and possibilities. Sex Educ. 2005;5(4):405–22.

313. Adamchak S. Youth peer education in reproductive health and HIV/AIDS. Youth issues paper 7. Arlington (VA): Family Health International/YouthNet; 2006.

314. Fischer S, Pedersen K, editors. Evidence-based guidelines for youth peer education. Research Triangle Park (VA): Family Health International; 2010.

315. Svenson G, Burke H. Formative research on peer education program productivity and sustainability. Youth research working paper No. 3. Arlington (VA): Family Health International/YouthNet; 2005.

316. Shepherd J, Peersman G, Weston R, Napuli I. Cervical cancer and sexual lifestyle: a systematic review of health education interventions targeted at women. Health Educ Res. 2000;15(6):681–94.

317. Jewkes R, Nduna M, Levin J, Jama N, Dunkle K, Puren A, et al. Impact of Stepping Stones on incidence of HIV and HSV-2 and sexual behaviour in rural South Africa: cluster randomised controlled trial. BMJ. 2008;337:a506.

318. Jewkes R, Wood K, Duvury N. "I woke up after I joined Stepping Stones": meanings of an HIV behavioural intervention in rural South African young people's lives. Health Educ Res. 2010;25(6):1074–84.

319. Wallace T. Evaluating Stepping Stones: a review of existing evaluations and ideas for future M&E work. Johannesburg: Action Aid; 2006.

320. Bianco M, Mariño A. EROTICs: an exploratory research on sexuality and the internet – policy review. Association for Progressive Communications, Women's Networking Support Program; 2008 (http://www.genderit.org/sites/default/upload/APCEROTICS_PolicyReview.pdf, accessed 5 February 2015).

321. The Siracusa Principles on the Limitation and Derogation Provisions in the International Covenant on Civil and Political Rights. New York (NY): United Nations Economic and Social Council; 1985 (E/CN.4/1985/4, Annex (1985)).

322. American Declaration of the Rights and Duties of Man. Washington (DC): Organization of American States; 1948.

323. American Convention on Human Rights. San José, Costa Rica: Organization of American States; 1969.

324. General comment No. 34: Freedoms of opinion and expression. Geneva: United Nations Human Rights Committee; 2011 (CCPR/C/GC/34).

325. Report of the Committee on the Elimination of Discrimination against Women. Twentieth session and twenty-first session. New York (NY): United Nations; 1999 (A/54/38/Rev.1 (Supp) Chapter IV. Consideration of reports submitted by States Parties under article 18 of the Convention. Section B.1. Initial periodic report of Kyrgyzstan).

326. Convention on the Elimination of All Forms of Discrimination against Women. New York (NY): United Nations; 1979.

327. African Union. Maputo plan of action for the operationalisation of the continental policy framework for sexual and reproductive health and rights 2007–2010. Addis Ababa: African Union; 2006 (AU Doc. Sp/MIN/CAMH/5(I)).

328. Ministers of Health and Education in Latin America and the Caribbean. Ministerial declaration: preventing through education. First meeting of Ministers of Health and Education to stop HIV and STIs in Latin America and the Caribbean, 1 August 2008, Mexico City.

329. *Lei n.º 3/84, de 24 de Março, Educação sexual e planeamento familiar* [Law No. 3/84 on sexual education and family planning]. Portugal; 1984 (in Portuguese).

330. *Lei n.º 60/2009 de 6 de Agosto, Estabelece o regime de aplicação da educação sexual em meio escolar* [Law No. 60/2009 on sexuality education]. Portugal; 2009 (in Portuguese).

331. *Caso Ríos y otros v. Venezuela (Excepciones preliminares, fondo, reparaciones y costas)*, decided on 28 January 2009. Washington (DC): Inter-American Court of Human Rights; 2009 (Series C No. 194).

332. Open Door and Dublin Well Woman v. Ireland. Application Nos. 14234/88 and 14235/88. Strasbourg: European Court of Human Rights; 1992.

333. HIV/AIDS Prevention and Control Act, No. 14 of 2006. Republic of Kenya; 2006.

334. The HIV/AIDS (Prevention and Control) Act. 2008. United Republic of Tanzania; 2008.

335. *Ley General para el Combate del Virus de Inmunodeficiencia Humana VIH y del Síndrome de Inmunodeficiencia Adquirida SIDA y de la promoción, protección y defensa de los Derechos Humanos ante el VIH-SIDA* [General Act on the Fight against HIV/AIDS and the Promotion, Protection, and Defense of Human Rights in the HIV/AIDS Field of Guatemala] Decreto 27-2000 [Decree 27-2000]. República de Guatemala; 2000 (in Spanish).

336. *Código penal federal* [Federal Penal Code]. Estados Unidos Mexicanos; 1931 (in Spanish).

337. Wellings K, Collumbien M, Slaymaker E, Singh S, Hodges Z, Patel D, et al. Sexual behaviour in context: a global perspective. Lancet. 2006;386(9548):1706–28.

338. European Social Charter. Council of Europe Treaty Series No. 35. Turin: Council of Europe; 1961.

339. African Charter on the Rights and Welfare of the Child. Addis Ababa: Organization of African Unity; 1990 (OAU Doc CAB/LEG/24.9/49 (1990)).

340. Kjeldsen, Busk Madsen and Pederson v. Denmark, Appl. Nos. 5095/71, 5920/72, 5926/72. Strasbourg: European Court of Human Rights; 1976.

341. *Sentencia No. T-440/92*, decided on 2 July 1992. República de Colombia Consejo de Estado [Council of State of the Republic of Colombia]; 1992 (in Spanish).

342. S*entencia No. T-337/95*, decided 26 July 1995. República de Colombia Consejo de Estado [Council of State of the Republic of Colombia]; 1995 (in Spanish).

343. S*entencia No. T-293/98*, decided 9 June 1998. República de Colombia Consejo de Estado [Council of State of the Republic of Colombia]; 1998 (in Spanish).

344. *Sentencia No. T-368/03*, decided 8 May 2003. República de Colombia Consejo de Estado [Council of State of the Republic of Colombia]; 2003 (in Spanish).

345. *Sentencia No. T-220/04*, decided 8 March 2004. República de Colombia Consejo de Estado [Council of State of the Republic of Colombia]; 2004 (in Spanish).

346. *Sentencia No. T-251/05*, decided 17 March 2005. República de Colombia Consejo de Estado [Council of State of the Republic of Colombia]; 2005 (in Spanish).

347. Krug EG, Dahlberg LL, Mercy JA, Zwi AB, Lozano R, editors. World report on violence and health. Geneva: World Health Organization; 2002.

348. García-Moreno C, Jansen HAFM, Ellsberg M, Heise L, Watts C. WHO Multi-country study on women's health and domestic violence against women. Initial results on prevalence, health outcomes and women's responses. Geneva: World Health Organization; 2005.

349. World Health Organization (WHO), London School of Hygiene and Tropical Medicine, South African Medical Research Council. Global and regional estimates of violence against women: prevalence and health effects of intimate partner violence and non-partner sexual violence against women. Geneva: WHO; 2013.

350. Jewkes R, Sen P, García-Moreno C. Sexual violence. In: Krug EG, Dahlberg LL, Mercy JA, Zwi AB, Lozano R, editors. World report on violence and health. Geneva: World Health Organization; 2002.

351. Campbell JC. Health consequences of intimate partner violence. Lancet. 2002;359:1331–6.

352. Plichta SB, Falik M. Prevalence of violence and its implications for women's health. Women's Health Issues. 2001;11:244–58.

353. Fonck K, Els L, Kidula N, Ndinya-Achola J, Temmerman M. Increased risk of HIV in women experiencing physical partner violence in Nairobi, Kenya. AIDS Behav. 2005;9:335–9.

354. Dunkle KL, Jewkes RK, Brown HC, Gray GE, McIntryre JA, Harlow SD. Gender-based violence, relationship power, and risk of HIV infection in women attending antenatal clinics in South Africa. Lancet. 2004;363:1415–21.

355. Maman S, Mbwambo JK, Hogan NM, Kilonzo GP, Campbell JC, Weiss E, Sweat MD. HIV-positive women report more lifetime partner violence: findings from a voluntary counseling and testing clinic in Dar es Salaam, Tanzania. Am J Public Health. 2002;92:1331–7.

356. Preventing intimate partner and sexual violence against women: taking action and generating evidence. Geneva: World Health Organization; 2010.

357. Violence against women. Fact sheet No. 239. Geneva: World Health Organization; updated 2014 (http://www.who.int/mediacentre/factsheets/fs239/en/index.html, accessed 5 February 2015).

358. Sokoloff NJ, Dupont I. Domestic violence at the intersections of race, class, and gender: challenges and contributions to understanding violence against marginalized women in diverse communities. Violence Against Women. 2005;11(1):38–64.

359. García-Moreno C, Watts C. Violence against women: an urgent public health priority. Bull World Health Organ. 2011;89:2.

360. Oosterhoff P, Zwanikken P, Ketting E. Sexual torture of men in Croatia and other conflict situations: an open secret. Reprod Health Matters. 2004;12(23):68–77.

361. Russell W. Sexual violence against men and boys. Forced Migr Rev. 2007;27:22–3.

362. Human Security Centre. Human Security Report 2005: War and peace in the 21st century. New York (NY): Oxford University Press; 2005.

307. Kirby D. Sex and HIV programs: their impact on sexual behaviors of young people throughout the world. J Adolesc Health. 2007;40:206–17.

308. Lazarus JV, Sihvonen-Riemenschneider H, Laukamm-Josten U, Wong F, Liljestrand J. Systematic review of interventions to prevent the spread of sexually transmitted infections, including HIV, among young people in Europe. Croat Med J. 2010;51(1):74–84.

309. Michielsen K, Chersich MF, Luchters S, De Koker P, Van Rossem R, Temmerman M. Effectiveness of HIV prevention for youth in sub-Saharan Africa: systematic review and meta-analysis of randomized and nonrandomized trials. AIDS. 2010;24(8):1193–202.

310. Oringanje C, Meremikwu MM, Eko H, Esu E, Meremikwu A, Ehiri JE. Interventions for preventing unintended pregnancies among adolescents. Cochrane Database Syst Rev. 2009;4. doi:10.1002/14651858.CD005215.pub2.

311. Robin L, Dittus P, Whitaker D, Crosby R, Ethier K, Mezoff J, et al. Behavioral interventions to reduce incidence of HIV, STD, and pregnancy among adolescents: a decade in review. J Adol Health. 2004;34(1):3–26.

312. Morris R. Research and evaluation in sexuality education: an allegorical exploration of complexities and possibilities. Sex Educ. 2005;5(4):405–22.

313. Adamchak S. Youth peer education in reproductive health and HIV/AIDS. Youth issues paper 7. Arlington (VA): Family Health International/YouthNet; 2006.

314. Fischer S, Pedersen K, editors. Evidence-based guidelines for youth peer education. Research Triangle Park (VA): Family Health International; 2010.

315. Svenson G, Burke H. Formative research on peer education program productivity and sustainability. Youth research working paper No. 3. Arlington (VA): Family Health International/YouthNet; 2005.

316. Shepherd J, Peersman G, Weston R, Napuli I. Cervical cancer and sexual lifestyle: a systematic review of health education interventions targeted at women. Health Educ Res. 2000;15(6):681–94.

317. Jewkes R, Nduna M, Levin J, Jama N, Dunkle K, Puren A, et al. Impact of Stepping Stones on incidence of HIV and HSV-2 and sexual behaviour in rural South Africa: cluster randomised controlled trial. BMJ. 2008;337:a506.

318. Jewkes R, Wood K, Duvury N. "I woke up after I joined Stepping Stones": meanings of an HIV behavioural intervention in rural South African young people's lives. Health Educ Res. 2010;25(6):1074–84.

319. Wallace T. Evaluating Stepping Stones: a review of existing evaluations and ideas for future M&E work. Johannesburg: Action Aid; 2006.

320. Bianco M, Mariño A. EROTICs: an exploratory research on sexuality and the internet – policy review. Association for Progressive Communications, Women's Networking Support Program; 2008 (http://www.genderit.org/sites/default/upload/APCEROTICS_PolicyReview.pdf, accessed 5 February 2015).

321. The Siracusa Principles on the Limitation and Derogation Provisions in the International Covenant on Civil and Political Rights. New York (NY): United Nations Economic and Social Council; 1985 (E/CN.4/1985/4, Annex (1985)).

322. American Declaration of the Rights and Duties of Man. Washington (DC): Organization of American States; 1948.

323. American Convention on Human Rights. San José, Costa Rica: Organization of American States; 1969.

324. General comment No. 34: Freedoms of opinion and expression. Geneva: United Nations Human Rights Committee; 2011 (CCPR/C/GC/34).

325. Report of the Committee on the Elimination of Discrimination against Women. Twentieth session and twenty-first session. New York (NY): United Nations; 1999 (A/54/38/Rev.1 (Supp) Chapter IV. Consideration of reports submitted by States Parties under article 18 of the Convention. Section B.1. Initial periodic report of Kyrgyzstan).

326. Convention on the Elimination of All Forms of Discrimination against Women. New York (NY): United Nations; 1979.

327. African Union. Maputo plan of action for the operationalisation of the continental policy framework for sexual and reproductive health and rights 2007–2010. Addis Ababa: African Union; 2006 (AU Doc. Sp/MIN/CAMH/5(I)).

328. Ministers of Health and Education in Latin America and the Caribbean. Ministerial declaration: preventing through education. First meeting of Ministers of Health and Education to stop HIV and STIs in Latin America and the Caribbean, 1 August 2008, Mexico City.

329. Lei n.º 3/84, de 24 de Março, Educação sexual e planeamento familiar [Law No. 3/84 on sexual education and family planning]. Portugal; 1984 (in Portuguese).

330. Lei n.º 60/2009 de 6 de Agosto, Estabelece o regime de aplicação da educação sexual em meio escolar [Law No. 60/2009 on sexuality education]. Portugal; 2009 (in Portuguese).

331. Caso Ríos y otros v. Venezuela (Excepciones preliminares, fondo, reparaciones y costas), decided on 28 January 2009. Washington (DC): Inter-American Court of Human Rights; 2009 (Series C No. 194).

332. Open Door and Dublin Well Woman v. Ireland. Application Nos. 14234/88 and 14235/88. Strasbourg: European Court of Human Rights; 1992.

363. General Comment No. 2: Implementation of Article 2 by States Parties. Geneva: United Nations Committee Against Torture; 2008 (CAT/C/GC/2).

364. Declaration on the elimination of violence against women. New York (NY): United Nations General Assembly; 1993.

365. Aydin v. Turkey. Application No. 23178/94, decided on 25 September 1997. Strasbourg: European Court of Human Rights; 1997.

366. Ana, Beatriz and Celia González v. Mexico, Case 11.565, Report No. 53/01 (Merits), decided on 4 April 2001. Washington (DC): Inter-American Commission on Human Rights; 2001 (OEA/Ser.L/V/II.111 Doc.20 rev. at 1097(2001)).

367. Caso Velasquez-Rodriguez v. Honduras, decided on 29 July 1988. San José, Costa Rica: Inter-American Court of Human Rights; 1988.

368. Heise L. What works to prevent partner violence: an evidence overview. London: STRIVE Research Consortium; 2011.

369. Caceres CF. Assessing young people's non-consensual sexual experiences: lessons from Peru. In: Jejeebhoy S, Shah I, Thapa S, editors. Sex without consent: young people in developing countries. London: Zed Books; 2005.

370. Caceres CF, Marin BV, Hudes ES, et al. Young people and the structure of sexual risks in Lima. AIDS. 1997;11(suppl.1):S67–77.

371. Erulkar AS. The experience of sexual coercion among young people in Kenya. Int Fam Plan Perspect. 2004;30(4):182–9.

372. Gupta A, Ailawadi A. Childhood and adolescent sexual abuse and incest: experiences of women survivors in India. In: Jejeebhoy S, Shah I, Thapa S, editors. Sex without consent: young people in developing countries. London: Zed Books; 2005.

373. Koenig MA, Zablotska I, Lutalo T, Nalugoda F, Wagman J, Gray R. Coerced first intercourse and reproductive health among adolescent women in Rakai, Uganda. In: Jejeebhoy S, Shah I, Thapa S, editors. Sex without consent: young people in developing countries. London: Zed Books; 2005.

374. Mpangile GS, Leshabari MT, Kihwele DJ. Induced abortion in Dar es Salaam, Tanzania: the plight of adolescents. In: Mundigo AI, Indriso C, editors. Abortion in the developing world. New Delhi: Vistaar Publications; 1999.

375. Mulugeta E, Kassaye, Berhane Y. Prevalence and outcomes of sexual violence among high school students. Ethiopian Med J. 1998;36:167–74.

376. Silberschmidt M, Rausch V. Adolescent girls, illegal abortions and "sugar-daddies" in Dar es Salaam: vulnerable victims and active social agents. Soc Sci Med. 2001;52:1815–26.

377. Worku A, Addisie M. Sexual violence among female high school students in Debark, north west Ethiopia. East Afr Med J. 2002;79(2):96–9.

378. Zierler S, Feingold L, Laufer D, Velentgas P, Kantrowitz-Gordon I, Mayer K. Adult survivors of childhood sexual abuse and subsequent risk of HIV infection. Am J Public Health. 1991;81(5):572–5.

379. Garner BA, editor. Black's Law Dictionary. Boston (MA): West Publishing Company; 2009.

380. Elements of crimes. The Hague: International Criminal Court, Assembly of States Parties; 2011 (Official Records ICC-PIDS-LT-03-002/11_Eng).

381. Report of the Committee on the Elimination of Discrimination against Women. Twenty-sixth and twenty-seventh session. New York (NY): United Nations; 2002 (A/57/38 (Supp). Chapter IV. Consideration of reports submitted by States Parties under article 18 of the Convention. Section B.4. Third and fourth period reports of Sri Lanka).

382. C.R. v. the United Kingdom. Application Nos. 20166/92 and 20190/92, decided on 22 November 1995. Strasbourg: European Court of Human Rights; 1995.

383. Criminal Code Amendment Act (No. 19) B.E. 2550, 2007. Social Division, Department of International Organizations, Ministry of Foreign Affairs, Kingdom of Thailand; 2007 (http://www.mfa.go.th/humanrights/implementation-of-un-resolutions/62-thailands-implementation-of-general-assembly-resolution-61143-, accessed 5 May 2014).

384. Criminal Law (Sexual Offences and Related Matters) Amendment Act, No. 32 of 2007. Republic of South Africa; 2007.

385. Rules of procedure and evidence. New York (NY): International Criminal Court, Assembly of States Parties; 2002 (Official Records ICC-ASP/1/3).

386. S v. J 1998 (4) BCLR 424. Republic of South Africa Supreme Court of Appeal; 1998.

387. Mukungu v. Republic (2003) AHRLR 175 (KeCA 2003). Republic of Kenya Court of Appeal; 2003.

388. National Prison Rape Elimination Commission Report. United States of America National Prison Rape Elimination Commission; 2009.

389. Consideration of reports submitted by States Parties under Article 19 of the Convention: Conclusions and recommendations of the Committee against Torture – United States of America. Second periodic report. Geneva: United Nations Committee against Torture; 2006 (CAT/C/USA/CO/2).

390. General Comment No. 2: Implementation of Article 2 by States Parties. Geneva: United Nations Committee Against Torture; 2007 (CAT/C/GC/2).

391. Stotzer RL. Comparison of hate crimes rates across protected and unprotected groups. Los Angeles (CA): The Williams Institute, UCLA School of Law; 2007.

392. Prison Rape Elimination Act of 2003, Public Law 108-79-SEPT. 4, 2003. United States of America Congress; 2003.

393. Child maltreatment. Fact sheet No. 150. Geneva: World Health Organization; 2010.

394. Jejeebhoy SJ, Bott S. Non-consensual sexual experiences of young people in developing countries: an overview. In: Jejeebhoy SJ, Shah I, Thapa S, editors. Sex without consent: young people in developing countries. London: Zed Books; 2005:3–45.

395. Child sexual abuse: a silent health emergency. WHO Regional Committee for Africa. Brazzaville: World Health Organization; 2004.

396. Boyer D, Fine D. Sexual abuse as a factor in adolescent pregnancy. Fam Plann Perspect. 1992;24:4–11.

397. Ellsberg MC. Sexual violence against women and girls: recent findings from Latin America and the Caribbean. In: Jejeebhoy S, Shah I, Thapa S, editors. Sex without consent: young people in developing countries. London: Zed Books; 2005.

398. Hanwerker WP. Gender power differences between parents and high-risk sexual behaviour by their children: AIDS/STD risk factors extend to a prior generation. J Womens Health.1993;2(3):301–16.

399. Heise L, Moore K, Toubia N. Sexual coercion and reproductive health: a focus on research. New York (NY): Population Council; 1995.

400. Somse P, Chapko MK, Hawkins RV. Multiple sexual partners: results of a national HIV/AIDS survey in the Central African Republic. AIDS. 1993;7(4):579–83.

401. Stewart L, Sebastiani A, Delgado G, López G. Consequences of sexual abuse of adolescents. Reprod Health Matters. 1996;4(7):129–34.

402. Council of Europe Convention on the protection of children against sexual exploitation and sexual abuse. Treaty Series No. 201. Lanzarote: Council of Europe; 2007.

403. Optional Protocol to the Convention on the Rights of the Child on the sale of children, child prostitution and child pornography. New York (NY): United Nations General Assembly; 2000 (Annex II).

404. Universal Declaration of Human Rights. New York (NY): United Nations; 1948.

405. Convention on Consent to Marriage, Minimum Age for Marriage and Registration of Marriages (1962). General Assembly resolution 1763 A (XVII) adopted 7 November 1962, entry into force 9 December 1964. New York (NY): United Nations; 1962.

406. Strengthening efforts to prevent and eliminate child, early and forced marriage: challenges, achievements, best practices and implementation gaps. Geneva: Human Rights Council; 2013.

407. Report of the Secretary General: Forced marriage of the girl child. New York (NY): United Nations Economic and Social Council; 2007.

408. Child Marriage Fact Sheet. New York (NY): United Nations Population Fund; 2005.

409. Early marriages, adolescent and young pregnancies. Report of the Secretariat. Sixty-Fifth World Health Assembly A65/13. Geneva: World Health Organization; 2012.

410. Clark S. Early marriage and HIV risks in sub-Saharan Africa. Stud Fam Plann. 2004;35(3):149–60.

411. Clark S, Bruce J, Dude A. Protecting young women from HIV(AIDS: the case against child and adolescent marriage. Int Fam Plan Perspect. 2006;32(2):79–88.

412. Borja J, Adair LS. Assessing the net effect of young maternal age on birthweight. Am J Hum Biol. 2003;15(6):733–40.

413. Choe MK, Thapa S, Mishra V. Early marriage and early motherhood in Nepal. J Biosoc Sci. 2005;37(2):142–62.

414. Keskinoglu P, Bilgic N, Picakciefe M, Giray H, Karakus N, Gunay T. Perinatal outcomes and risk factors of Turkish adolescent mothers. J Pediatr Adolesc Gynecol. 2007;20(1):19–24.

415. Koniak-Griffin D, Turner-Pluta C. Health risks and psychosocial outcomes of early childbearing: a review of the literature. J Perinat Neonatal Nurs. 2001;15(2):1–17.

416. Raj A, Saggurti N, Winter M, Labonte A, Decker MR, Salaiah D, Silverman JG. The effect of maternal child marriage on morbidity and mortality of children under 5 in India: cross sectional study of a nationally representative sample. BMJ. 2010;340:b4258.

417. Shawky S, Milaat W. Cumulative impact of early maternal marital age during the childbearing period. Peaediatr Perinat Ep. 2001;15(1):27–33.

418. Senderowitz J. Adolescent health: Reassessing the passage to adulthood. World Bank Discussion Paper No. 272. Washington (DC): World Bank; 1995.

419. Early marriage, child spouses. Innocenti Digest No. 7. Florence: United Nations Children's Fund; 2001.

390. General Comment No. 2: Implementation of Article 2 by States Parties. Geneva: United Nations Committee Against Torture; 2007 (CAT/C/GC/2).

391. Stotzer RL. Comparison of hate crimes rates across protected and unprotected groups. Los Angeles (CA): The Williams Institute, UCLA School of Law; 2007.

392. Prison Rape Elimination Act of 2003, Public Law 108-79-SEPT. 4, 2003. United States of America Congress; 2003.

393. Child maltreatment. Fact sheet No. 150. Geneva: World Health Organization; 2010.

394. Jejeebhoy SJ, Bott S. Non-consensual sexual experiences of young people in developing countries: an overview. In: Jejeebhoy SJ, Shah I, Thapa S, editors. Sex without consent: young people in developing countries. London: Zed Books; 2005:3–45.

395. Child sexual abuse: a silent health emergency. WHO Regional Committee for Africa. Brazzaville: World Health Organization; 2004.

396. Boyer D, Fine D. Sexual abuse as a factor in adolescent pregnancy. Fam Plann Perspect. 1992;24:4–11.

397. Ellsberg MC. Sexual violence against women and girls: recent findings from Latin America and the Caribbean. In: Jejeebhoy S, Shah I, Thapa S, editors. Sex without consent: young people in developing countries. London: Zed Books; 2005.

398. Hanwerker WP. Gender power differences between parents and high-risk sexual behaviour by their children: AIDS/STD risk factors extend to a prior generation. J Womens Health.1993;2(3):301–16.

399. Heise L, Moore K, Toubia N. Sexual coercion and reproductive health: a focus on research. New York (NY): Population Council; 1995.

400. Somse P, Chapko MK, Hawkins RV. Multiple sexual partners: results of a national HIV/AIDS survey in the Central African Republic. AIDS. 1993;7(4):579–83.

401. Stewart L, Sebastiani A, Delgado G, López G. Consequences of sexual abuse of adolescents. Reprod Health Matters. 1996;4(7):129–34.

402. Council of Europe Convention on the protection of children against sexual exploitation and sexual abuse. Treaty Series No. 201. Lanzarote: Council of Europe; 2007.

403. Optional Protocol to the Convention on the Rights of the Child on the sale of children, child prostitution and child pornography. New York (NY): United Nations General Assembly; 2000 (Annex II).

404. Universal Declaration of Human Rights. New York (NY): United Nations; 1948.

405. Convention on Consent to Marriage, Minimum Age for Marriage and Registration of Marriages (1962). General Assembly resolution 1763 A (XVII) adopted 7 November 1962, entry into force 9 December 1964. New York (NY): United Nations; 1962.

406. Strengthening efforts to prevent and eliminate child, early and forced marriage: challenges, achievements, best practices and implementation gaps. Geneva: Human Rights Council; 2013.

407. Report of the Secretary General: Forced marriage of the girl child. New York (NY): United Nations Economic and Social Council; 2007.

408. Child Marriage Fact Sheet. New York (NY): United Nations Population Fund; 2005.

409. Early marriages, adolescent and young pregnancies. Report of the Secretariat. Sixty-Fifth World Health Assembly A65/13. Geneva: World Health Organization; 2012.

410. Clark S. Early marriage and HIV risks in sub-Saharan Africa. Stud Fam Plann. 2004;35(3):149–60.

411. Clark S, Bruce J, Dude A. Protecting young women from HIV(AIDS: the case against child and adolescent marriage. Int Fam Plan Perspect. 2006;32(2):79–88.

412. Borja J, Adair LS. Assessing the net effect of young maternal age on birthweight. Am J Hum Biol. 2003;15(6):733–40.

413. Choe MK, Thapa S, Mishra V. Early marriage and early motherhood in Nepal. J Biosoc Sci. 2005;37(2):142–62.

414. Keskinoglu P, Bilgic N, Picakciefe M, Giray H, Karakus N, Gunay T. Perinatal outcomes and risk factors of Turkish adolescent mothers. J Pediatr Adolesc Gynecol. 2007;20(1):19–24.

415. Koniak-Griffin D, Turner-Pluta C. Health risks and psychosocial outcomes of early childbearing: a review of the literature. J Perinat Neonatal Nurs. 2001;15(2):1–17.

416. Raj A, Saggurti N, Winter M, Labonte A, Decker MR, Salaiah D, Silverman JG. The effect of maternal child marriage on morbidity and mortality of children under 5 in India: cross sectional study of a nationally representative sample. BMJ. 2010;340:b4258.

417. Shawky S, Milaat W. Cumulative impact of early maternal marital age during the childbearing period. Peaediatr Perinat Ep. 2001;15(1):27–33.

418. Senderowitz J. Adolescent health: Reassessing the passage to adulthood. World Bank Discussion Paper No. 272. Washington (DC): World Bank; 1995.

419. Early marriage, child spouses. Innocenti Digest No. 7. Florence: United Nations Children's Fund; 2001.

363. General Comment No. 2: Implementation of Article 2 by States Parties. Geneva: United Nations Committee Against Torture; 2008 (CAT/C/GC/2).

364. Declaration on the elimination of violence against women. New York (NY): United Nations General Assembly; 1993.

365. Aydin v. Turkey. Application No. 23178/94, decided on 25 September 1997. Strasbourg: European Court of Human Rights; 1997.

366. Ana, Beatriz and Celia González v. Mexico, Case 11.565, Report No. 53/01 (Merits), decided on 4 April 2001. Washington (DC): Inter-American Commission on Human Rights; 2001 (OEA/Ser.L/V/II.111 Doc.20 rev. at 1097(2001)).

367. Caso Velasquez-Rodriguez v. Honduras, decided on 29 July 1988. San José, Costa Rica: Inter-American Court of Human Rights; 1988.

368. Heise L. What works to prevent partner violence: an evidence overview. London: STRIVE Research Consortium; 2011.

369. Caceres CF. Assessing young people's non-consensual sexual experiences: lessons from Peru. In: Jejeebhoy S, Shah I, Thapa S, editors. Sex without consent: young people in developing countries. London: Zed Books; 2005.

370. Caceres CF, Marin BV, Hudes ES, et al. Young people and the structure of sexual risks in Lima. AIDS. 1997;11(suppl.1):S67–77.

371. Erulkar AS. The experience of sexual coercion among young people in Kenya. Int Fam Plan Perspect. 2004;30(4):182–9.

372. Gupta A, Ailawadi A. Childhood and adolescent sexual abuse and incest: experiences of women survivors in India. In: Jejeebhoy S, Shah I, Thapa S, editors. Sex without consent: young people in developing countries. London: Zed Books; 2005.

373. Koenig MA, Zablotska I, Lutalo T, Nalugoda F, Wagman J, Gray R. Coerced first intercourse and reproductive health among adolescent women in Rakai, Uganda. In: Jejeebhoy S, Shah I, Thapa S, editors. Sex without consent: young people in developing countries. London: Zed Books; 2005.

374. Mpangile GS, Leshabari MT, Kihwele DJ. Induced abortion in Dar es Salaam, Tanzania: the plight of adolescents. In: Mundigo AI, Indriso C, editors. Abortion in the developing world. New Delhi: Vistaar Publications; 1999.

375. Mulugeta E, Kassaye, Berhane Y. Prevalence and outcomes of sexual violence among high school students. Ethiopian Med J. 1998;36:167–74.

376. Silberschmidt M, Rausch V. Adolescent girls, illegal abortions and "sugar-daddies" in Dar es Salaam: vulnerable victims and active social agents. Soc Sci Med. 2001;52:1815–26.

377. Worku A, Addisie M. Sexual violence among female high school students in Debark, north west Ethiopia. East Afr Med J. 2002;79(2):96–9.

378. Zierler S, Feingold L, Laufer D, Velentgas P, Kantrowitz-Gordon I, Mayer K. Adult survivors of childhood sexual abuse and subsequent risk of HIV infection. Am J Public Health. 1991;81(5):572–5.

379. Garner BA, editor. Black's Law Dictionary. Boston (MA): West Publishing Company; 2009.

380. Elements of crimes. The Hague: International Criminal Court, Assembly of States Parties; 2011 (Official Records ICC-PIDS-LT-03-002/11_Eng).

381. Report of the Committee on the Elimination of Discrimination against Women. Twenty-sixth and twenty-seventh session. New York (NY): United Nations; 2002 (A/57/38 (Supp). Chapter IV. Consideration of reports submitted by States Parties under article 18 of the Convention. Section B.4. Third and fourth period reports of Sri Lanka).

382. C.R. v. the United Kingdom. Application Nos. 20166/92 and 20190/92, decided on 22 November 1995. Strasbourg: European Court of Human Rights; 1995.

383. Criminal Code Amendment Act (No. 19) B.E. 2550, 2007. Social Division, Department of International Organizations, Ministry of Foreign Affairs, Kingdom of Thailand; 2007 (http://www.mfa.go.th/humanrights/implementation-of-un-resolutions/62-thailands-implementation-of-general-assembly-resolution-61143-, accessed 5 May 2014).

384. Criminal Law (Sexual Offences and Related Matters) Amendment Act, No. 32 of 2007. Republic of South Africa; 2007.

385. Rules of procedure and evidence. New York (NY): International Criminal Court, Assembly of States Parties; 2002 (Official Records ICC-ASP/1/3).

386. S v. J 1998 (4) BCLR 424. Republic of South Africa Supreme Court of Appeal; 1998.

387. Mukungu v. Republic (2003) AHRLR 175 (KeCA 2003). Republic of Kenya Court of Appeal; 2003.

388. National Prison Rape Elimination Commission Report. United States of America National Prison Rape Elimination Commission; 2009.

389. Consideration of reports submitted by States Parties under Article 19 of the Convention: Conclusions and recommendations of the Committee against Torture – United States of America. Second periodic report. Geneva: United Nations Committee against Torture; 2006 (CAT/C/USA/CO/2).

420. Conde-Agudelo A, Belizan JM, Lammers C. Maternal-perinatal morbidity and mortality associated with adolescent pregnancy in Latin America: cross-sectional study. Am J Obstet Gynecol. 2005;192(2):342–9.

421. Resolution adopted by the General Assembly 60/141. The girl child. New York (NY): United Nations General Assembly; 2006.

422. Case No. 255711, heard 21 February 2001. Algerian Supreme Court; 2001.

423. Karimotu Yakubu v. Alhaji Paiko, CA/K/80s/85. Kaduna State, Nigeria: Federal Republic of Nigeria Court of Appeal; 1985.

424. Prosecutor v. Alex Tamba Brima, Brima Bazzy Kamara and Santigie Borbor Kanu. Appeals Chamber of the Special Court for Sierra Leone; 2008 (http://www.refworld.org/docid/467fba742.html, accessed 5 February 2015).

425. Agarwal B. A field of one's own: gender and land rights in South Asia. Cambridge: Cambridge University Press; 1995.

426. Banda F. Women, law and human rights: an African perspective. Portland (OR): Hart Publishing; 2005.

427. Ewelukwa UU. Post-colonialism, gender, customary injustice: widows in African societies. Hum Rights Quart. 2002;24(2):424–86.

428. Understanding and addressing violence against women. Geneva: World Health Organization; 2012.

429. Supplementary Convention on the Abolition of Slavery, the Slave Trade, and Institutions and Practices Similar to Slavery. Geneva: United Nations Economic and Social Council; 1956.

430. The Criminal Code: Federal Negarit Gazeta under Proclamation No. 414/2004, came into force as of 9 May 2005. Federal Democratic Republic of Ethiopia; 2004.

431. Hate crimes in the OSCE region – incidents and responses. Annual Report for 2006. Warsaw: Organization for Security and Cooperation in Europe/Office for Democratic Institutions and Human Rights; 2007.

432. Trans murder monitoring project reveals more than 800 reported murders of trans people in the last four years. Press release March 2012. Transgender Europe; 2012 (http://www.tgeu.org/node/290, accessed 5 February 2015).

433. Sandfort TG, Melendez RM, Diaz RM. Gender nonconformity, homophobia, and mental distress in Latino gay and bisexual men. J Sex Res. 2007;44(2):181–9.

434. Human rights, sexual orientation and gender identity. Washington (DC): Organization of American States; 2013 (OAS/AG/RES.2653 (XLI-O/11)).

435. Lombardi EL, Wilchins RA, Priesing D, Malouf D. Gender violence: transgender experiences with violence and discrimination. J Homosex. 2001;42(1):89–101.

436. Lahir A. Vulnerability of male and transgender sex workers to STIs/HIV in the context of violence and other human rights violations. Presentation given at the 8th International Congress on AIDS in Asia and the Pacific, Sri Lanka, 2007.

437. Moradian A. The complexities of human sexuality, and Islamic laws and regulations in Iran. Chicago (IL): The Chicago School of Professional Psychology; 2009.

438. Concluding observations: Poland. New York (NY): United Nations Committee on Economic, Social and Cultural Rights; 2009 (E/C.12/POL/CO/5).

439. Resolution adopted by the Human Rights Council. Human rights, sexual orientation and gender identity. New York (NY): United Nations General Assembly; 2014.

440. Resolution 1728 (2010): Discrimination on the basis of sexual orientation and gender identity. Strasbourg: Council of Europe Parliamentary Assembly; 2010.

441. Sentencing Act No. 49 of 1991. State of Victoria, Commonwealth of Australia; 1991.

442. Matthew Shepard and James Byrd, Jr., Hate Crimes Prevention Act of 2009, 18 U.S.C. § 249. United States Department of Justice; 2009.

443. The Law on the Prohibition of Discrimination [Unofficial translation from Serbian by Labris Serbia]. Serbia; 2009.

444. In-depth study on all forms of violence against women. Report of the Secretary-General. New York (NY): United Nations General Assembly; 2006.

445. Report of the Special Rapporteur on violence against women, its causes and consequences, Yakin Ertürk. Addendum: Mission to Turkey. Geneva: United Nations Human Rights Council; 2007.

446. Report of the Special Rapporteur on violence against women, its causes and consequences, Yakin Ertürk. Addendum: Mission to Sweden. Geneva: United Nations; 2007.

447. They want us exterminated: murder, torture, sexual orientation and gender in Iraq. Human Rights Watch Report 17 August 2009. New York (NY): Human Rights Watch; 2009.

448. The state of the world population: Chapter 3: ending violence against women and girls. New York (NY): United Nations Population Fund; 2000.

449. Turkish Penal Code, Law No. 5237. Republic of Turkey; 2004.

450. Convention relating to the Status of Refugees. New York (NY): United Nations; 1951.

451. UNHCR guidance note on refugee claims relating to sexual orientation and gender identity. Geneva: United Nations High Commissioner for Refugees; 2008.

452. Council Directive 2004/83/EC of 29 April 2004 on minimum standards for the qualification and status of third country nationals or stateless persons as refugees or as persons who otherwise need international protection and the content of the protection granted (Official Journal L304/12). European Union; 2004.

453. Geovanni Hernandez-Montiel v. INS, 225 F.3d 1084, decided on 24 August 2000. United States of America, Court of Appeals for the 9th Circuit; 2000.

454. Deering KN, Amin A, Shoveller J, Nesbitt A, Garcia-Moreno C, Duff P, et al. A systematic review of the correlates of violence against sex workers. Am J Public Health. 2014;104(5):e42–54. doi:10.2105/AJPH.2014.301909.

455. Church S, Henderson M, Barnard M, Hart G. Violence by clients towards female prostitutes in different work settings: questionnaire survey. BMJ. 2001;322:524–5.

456. Panchanadeswaran S, Johnson SS, Srikrishnan AK, Zelaya Ca, Solomon S, Go VF, Celentano D. A descriptive profile of abused female sex workers in India. J Health Popul Nutr. 2010;28(3):211–20.

457. Rhodes T, Simic M, Baros S, Platt. L, Zikic B. Police violence and sexual risk among female and transvestite sex workers in Serbia: a qualitative study. BMJ. 2008;337;a811.

458. Violence against sex workers and HIV prevention. Information Bulletin Series No. 3. Geneva: World Health Organization and The Global Coalition on Women and AIDS; 2005.

459. Gould C, Fick N. Selling sex in Cape Town: sex work and human trafficking in a South African city. Pretoria: Institute for Security Studies (ISS) and Sex Worker Education and Advocacy Taskforce (SWEAT); 2008.

460. Allinot S, Boer J, Brunemeyer N, Capler R, Cristen Gleeson DJ, Jacox K, et al. Voices for dignity: a call to end the harms caused by Canada's sex trade laws. Pivot Legal Society Sex Work Subcommittee; 2004.

461. Blankenship KM, Koester S. Criminal law, policing policy, and HIV risk in female street sex workers and injection drug users. J Law Med Ethics. 2002;30(4):548–59.

462. Crago AL, Rakhmetova A, Klaradafov M. Islamova S, Maslove I. Central and Eastern Europe and Central Asia: police raids and violence put sex workers at risk of HIV. HIV/AIDS Policy Law Rev. 2008;13(2-3):71–2.

463. Mayhew S, Collumbien M, Qureshi A, Platt L, Rafiq N, Faisel A, et al. Protecting the unprotected: mixed-method research on drug use, sex work and rights in Pakistan's fight against HIV/AIDS. Sex Transm Infect. 2009;85(Suppl 2):ii31–6.

464. Ngo Anh D, McCurdy SA, Ross MW, Markham C, Ratliff EA, Pham Hang TB. The lives of female sex workers in Vietnam: findings from a qualitative study. Cult Health Sex. 2007;9(6):555–70.

465. Jeffrey LA, Sullivan B. Canadian sex work policy for the 21st century: Enhancing rights and safety, lessons from Australia. Can Pol Sci Rev. 2009;3(1):57–76.

466. Karandikar S, Moises P. From client to pimp: male violence against female sex workers. J Interpers Violence. 2010;25:257–73.

467. Lutnick A, Cohan D. Criminalization, legalization or decriminalization of sex work: what female sex workers say in San Francisco, USA. Reprod Health Matters. 2009;17(34):38–46.

468. Miller J. Violence and coercion in Sri Lanka's commercial sex industry. Violence Against Women. 2002;8:1044–73.

469. Memorandum of support for New York State Bill S.323/A.1008. Ending the use of condom possession as evidence of prostitution. New York (NY): Human Rights Watch; 2012.

470. Wurth MH, Schleifer, McLemore M, Todrys KW, Amon JJ. Condoms as evidence of prostitution in the United States and the criminalization of sex work. J Int AIDS Soc. 2013;16(1):10.7448/IAS.

471. Alexander P. Sex work and health: a question of safety in the workplace. J Am Med Womens Assoc. 1998;53(2):77–82.

472. Shannon K Strathdee SA, Shoveller J, Rusch M, Kerr T, Tyndall MW. Structural and environmental barriers to condom use negotiation with clients among female sex workers: implications for HIV-prevention strategies and policy. Am J Public Health. 2009;99(4):659–65.

473. Pitcher J, Campbell R, Hubbard P, O'Beill M, Scoular J. Living and working in areas of street sex work: from conflict to coexistence. York, United Kingdom: Joseph Rowntree Foundation and The Policy Press; 2006.

474. Yi H, Mantell JE, Wu R, Lu Z, Zeng J, Wan Y. A profile of HIV risk factors in the context of sex work environments among migrant female sex workers in Beijing, China. Psychol Health Med. 2010;15(2):172–87.

475. Brents BG, Hausbeck K. Violence and legalized brothel prostitution in Nevada: examining safety, risk and prostitution policy. J Interpers Violence. 2005;20(3):270–95.

476. Seib C, Fischer J, Najman JM. The health of female sex workers from three industry sectors in Queensland, Australia. Soc Sci Med. 2009;68:473–8.

477. Regulating prostitution: an evaluation of the Prostitution Act 1999 (QLD). Australia: Queensland Crime and Misconduct Commission; 2004.

478. Operating a licensed sex work business: guide for licensees and approved managers. Melbourne, Australia: Victorian Consumer and Business Center; 2001.

479. Trafficking in persons: global patterns. Vienna: United Nations Office on Drugs and Crime; 2006.

480. Gupta J, Raj A, Decker MR, Reed E, Silverman JG. HIV vulnerabilities of sex-trafficked Indian women and girls. Int J Gynaecol Obstet. 2009;107(1):30–4.

481. Silverman JG, Decker MR, Gupta J, Maheshwari A, Willis BM, Raj A. HIV prevalence and predicgtors of infection in sex-trafficked Nepalese girls and women. JAMA. 2007;298(5):536–42.

482. Zimmerman C, Hossain M, Yun K, Roche B, Morison L, Watts C. Stolen smiles: the physical and psychological health consequences of women and adolescents trafficked in Europe. London: London School of Hygiene and Tropical Medicine and The European Commission's Daphne Programme; 2006.

483. Zimmerman C, Hossain M, Yun K, Gajdadziev V, Guzun N, Tchomarova M, et al. The health of trafficked women: a survey of women entering posttrafficking services in Europe. Am J Public Health. 2008;98(1):55–9.

484. Zimmerman C, Kiss L, Hossain M, Watts C. Trafficking in persons: a health concern? Cien Saude Colet. 2009;14(4):1029–35.

485. Anti-Trafficking in Persons Act B.E. 2551 (2008). Kingdom of Thailand; 2008.

486. Recommended principles on human rights and human trafficking. Geneva: Office of the United Nations High Commissioner for Human Rights; 2002 (E/2002/68/Add.1).

487. Recommended Principles and Guidelines on Human Rights and Human Trafficking. New York (NY): United Nations Economic and Social Council; 2002.

488. Council of Europe Convention on action against trafficking in human beings. Council of Europe Treaty Series No. 197. Warsaw: Council of Europe; 2005.

489. Report of the Special Rapporteur on trafficking in persons, especially women and children Joy Ngozi Ezeilo. Geneva: United Nations Human Rights Council; 2011.

490. The state of the world's children 2012. New York (NY): United Nations Children's Fund; 2012.

491. Chalmers B, Hashi KO. 432 Somali women's birth experiences in Canada after earlier female genital mutilation. Birth. 2000;27:227–34.

492. Talle A. Female circumcision in Africa and beyond: the anthropology of a difficult issue. In: Hernlund Y, Shell-Duncan B, editors. Transcultural bodies: female genital cutting in global context. New Brunswick: Rutgers University Press; 2007:91–106.

493. Berg R, Denison E. Does female genital mutilation/cutting (FGM/C) affect women's sexual functioning? A systematic review of the sexual consequences of FGM/C. Sex Res Social Policy. 2012;9(1):41–56.

494. Berggren V, Yagoub AE, Satti AM, Khalifa MA, Aziz FA, Bergstrom S. Postpartum tightening operations on two delivering wards in Sudan. Br J Midwifery. 2006;14:1–4.

495. Gruenbaum E. Sexuality issues in the movement to abolish female genital cutting in Sudan. Med Anthropol Q. 2006;20:121.

496. Talle A. Transforming women into "pure" agnates: aspects of female infibulation in Somalia. In: Broch-Due V, Rudie I, Bleie T, editors. Carved flesh, cast selves: gender symbols and social practices. Oxford: Berg;1993:83–106.

497. Abusharaf RM. Virtuous cuts: female genital circumcision an African ontology. Differences, a Journal of Feminist Cultural Studies. 2001;12:112–40.

498. Ahmadu F. Rites and wrongs: an insider/outsider reflects on power and excision. In: Shell-Duncan B, Hernlund Y, editors. Female "circumcision" in Africa: culture, controversy and change. Boulder (CO): Lynne Rienner; 2000.

499. Hernlund Y. Cutting without ritual and ritual without cutting: female circumcision and the re-ritualization of initiation in the Gambia. In: Hernlund Y, Shell-Duncan B, editors. Female "circumcision" in Africa: culture, change and controversy. Boulder (CO): Lynne Rienner; 2000:235–52.

500. Johansen REB. Experiencing sex in exile: can genitals change their gender? In: Hernlund Y, Shell-Duncan B, editors. Transcultural bodies: female genital cutting in global context. New Brunswick: Rutgers University Press; 2007:248–77.

501. Almroth L, Almroth-Berggren V, Hassanein OM, Al-Said SS, Hasan SS, Lithell UB, et al. Male complications of female genital mutilation. Soc Sci Med. 2001;53:1455–60. doi:10.1016/S0277-9536(00)00428-7.

502. General Recommendation No. 14: Female circumcision. New York (NY): United Nations Committee on the Elimination of Discrimination against Women; 1990 (A/45/38).

503. Protocol on gender and development of the Southern African Development Community. Johannesburg: Southern African Development Community; 2008.

504. Global strategy to stop health-care providers from performing female genital mutilation. Geneva: World Health Organization; 2010.

505. Legislative reform to support the abandonment of female genital mutilation/cutting. New York (NY): United Nations Children's Fund; 2010.

506. Kim Y. Asylum law and female genital mutilation: recent developments. CRS Report for Congress. Washington (DC): Congressional Research Service; 2008.

507. Executive Office for Immigration Review, Board of Immigration Appeals. Matter of S-A-K and H-A.H-, Respondents. Washington (DC): United States Department of Justice; 2008 (24 I&D Dec. 464 (BIA 2008)).

508. Cottingham J, Germain A, Hunt P. Use of human rights to meet the unmet need for family planning. Lancet. 2012;380:172–80.

509. Guidelines on ethical issues in the management of severely disabled women with gynecological problems. London: International Federation of Gynaecology and Obstetrics; 2011.

510. WMA statement on forced and coerced sterilisation. Adopted by 63rd WMA General Assembly, Bangkok Thailand, October 2012. World Medical Association (WMA); 2012 (http://www.wma.net/ en/30publications/10policies/s21/index.html, accessed 5 February 2015).

511. General Comment No. 13: The right of the child to freedom from all forms of violence. Geneva: United Nations Committee on the Rights of the Child; 2011 (CRC/C/GC/13).

512. Report of the Special Rapporteur on violence against women, its causes and consequences, Ms Radhika Coomaraswamy. Addendum 4: Policies and practices that impact women's reproductive rights and contribute to, cause or constitute violence against women. New York (NY): United Nations Commission on Human Rights; 1999.

513. General Comment No. 16: The equal right of men and women to the enjoyment of all economic, social and cultural rights. New York (NY): United Nations Committee on Economic, Social and Cultural Rights; 2005 (E/C.12/2005/4).

514. Concluding Observations: Spain. Geneva: United Nations Committee on the Rights of Persons with Disabilities; 2011 (CRPD/C/ESP/CO/1).

515. Concluding Observations: Argentina. Geneva: United Nations Committee on the Rights of Persons with Disabilities; 2012 (CRPD/C/ARG/CO/1).

516. Concluding Observations: China. Geneva: United Nations Committee on the Rights of Persons with Disabilities; 2012 (CRPD/C/CHN/CO/1).

517. Concluding Observations: Hungary. Geneva: United Nations Committee on the Rights of Persons with Disabilities; 2012 (CRPD/C/HUN/CO/1).

518. Concluding Observations: Peru. Geneva: United Nations Committee on the Rights of Persons with Disabilities; 2012 (CRPD/C/Per/CO/1).

519. Interim report of the Special Rapporteur on Torture and Other Cruel, Inhuman or Degrading Treatment or Punishment, Manfred Nowak. New York (NY): United Nations; 2008.

520. Baldizzone T, Baldizzone G. Wedding ceremonies: ethnic symbols, costume and rituals. Paris: Flammarion; 2001.

521. Concluding Observations: Combined third and fourth periodic report of Jordan. Geneva: United Nations Committee on the Elimination of Discrimination against Women; 2007 (CEDAW/C/JOR/CO/4).

522. Concluding Observations of the Committee on the Elimination of Discrimination against Women: South Africa. Combined second, third and fourth periodic reports. Geneva: United Nations Committee on the Elimination of Discrimination against Women; 2011 (CEDAW/C/ZAF/CO/4).

523. Supreme Court of Nepal. NKP 2055 (1998) vol. 8, p. 476. Cited in: Chagai RP. Judicial response to reproductive rights: experience of public interest litigation in Nepal. J Health Stud. 2008;I(2):24–47.